ELLE

GLAM FITNESS

COMPLETE CARDIO

ELLE

GLAM FITNESS
COMPLETE CARDIO

BY MELYSSA ST. MICHAEL, DONALD KASEN
AND DANIELLE KASEN

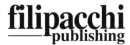

filipacchi
publishing

CONTENTS

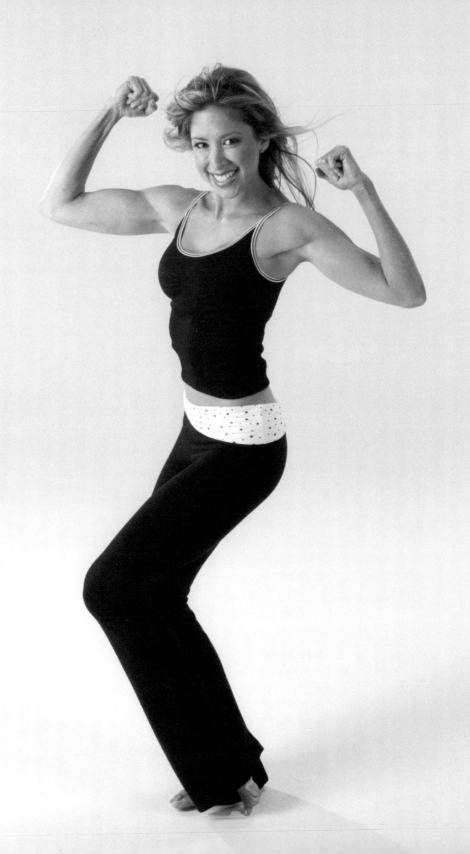

CHAPTER 1
CARDIO DANCE BASICS

Dance is not just fun; it's also great cardio exercise. Before you get grooving with ELLE's Glam Fitness Complete Cardio workout, take a few minutes to read on and learn the key points about cardio exercise that will not only make your workout fun, but safe and effective too.

In this chapter you will learn:

- what cardio exercise is;

- how cardio exercise improves your health;

- the different styles of dance;

- why dance exercise benefits your body;

- how to develop your mind-body connection.

THE CARDIO CONNECTION

If you have found your mid-section rolling over the top of your low-riders recently, you may have had well-meaning friends suggest crunches to whittle away your waist. Jiggly thighs? Leg lifts will firm and tone, they said. But when you crunched and lifted, and lifted and crunched, not one ounce of fat was burned off. So, why didn't your crunches and leg lifts work?

That's because to burn fat, you need to do cardio, or aerobic, exercise. By definition, aerobic exercise is any type of activity that uses the body's large muscle groups (such as your leg muscles) in a continuous, movement-oriented manner that keeps the heart rate and respiration elevated for a sustained period of time. Activities such as bike riding, walking, jogging, swimming and yes, you guessed it — cardio dance — fit the bill for aerobic exercise.

Cardio exercise does more than just help you to peel off the pounds. It also:

- strengthens your heart, lungs and circulatory system;
- helps reduce the risk of heart attacks, diabetes, high cholesterol, and high blood pressure;
- tones your muscles;
- increases your lung capacity so you can walk up three flights of stairs without huffing and puffing, or hold your breath for a very long time underwater;
- helps you sleep better;
- reduces stress;

- boosts your mood: feel-good chemicals called endorphins are released in the brain during long, continuous workouts that are moderate to high intensity.

To stay healthy, the recommended amount of cardio activity is 30 to 60 minutes per day, most days of the week. However, if just saying the word cardio makes you break a sweat, then any amount of cardio that you do will be a good amount of cardio, be it 15 minutes or 45 seconds. (More on that in Chapter 2, where we'll show you how to plan your first few workouts, gradually increasing the duration and intensity of your cardio dance workout as you become more conditioned.) Our goal for you right now is to just get you moving, and have fun while you are doing it.

WHAT'S THE DEAL ON DANCE?

The cardio dance moves in the ELLE Glam Dance Cardio Workout have their roots in such dance traditions as modern dance, ballet, ballroom, and hip hop.

MODERN DANCE

It's a form of dance where no two movements seem the same, and the dancer's movements are free and fluid. Modern dance was created in the early 20th century, and may have begun as a revolt against the rigid constraints of classical ballet. It's an expressive type of dancing; for example, if you're trying to express sadness, you would use slow movements.

BALLET

Ballet is a form of classical dance developed in the courts of Renaissance Italy that often (but not always) tells a story. Ballet has very particular rules about how the dancer must move; five basic positions serve as a foundation for more complicated ballet steps. When you do ballet moves, posture is important; for example, you want to keep your neck elongated and your rear tucked in.

HIP HOP

Popping, locking, break dancing, krumping — these are all forms of hip hop, a street dance style that originated in New York City in the 1970s. Hip hop is expressive and improvisational, and the styles vary widely. For example, break dancing has many ground moves while newer styles like krumping are performed in an upright position.

BALLROOM

From the improvisational West Coast Swing to the sexy tango, ballroom is a type of partner dance where two dancers, a leader and a follower, dance with physical contact through their upper bodies, lower bodies, or arms only. The dancers are typically on a crowded floor, which means they need to dance in synchrony without bumping into other dancers.

THE DANCE ADVANTAGE

Why dance? Why not step aerobics or swimming? Because dance offers a collection of health benefits that no other form of cardio exercise can match.

Cardio dance increases your heart rate, which makes your heart stronger and burns calories. You control the tempo of the exercise, so you'll never feel like your heart is about to pound right out of your chest!

Cardio dance increases your flexibility because it stretches all the muscles and joints through their natural ranges of motion. Being flexible means you can reach for a box on a top shelf or bend over to lace your shoes without feeling restricted or risking injury.

Cardio dance is a weight-bearing exercise — meaning you work your bones and muscles against gravity, unlike with swimming or cycling — and this is important for keeping bones strong. This type of exercise stimulates bone formation, and it also strengthens the muscles that pull on bones, which makes the bones stronger in response. Weight-bearing exercise like cardio dance also works your muscles, which means you'll not only become stronger you'll also look more toned. Have you heard of the "skinny fat" —people who are within their normal weight range but still flabby? That won't be you.

Say goodbye to klutziness — cardio dance ups your balance and coordination, thanks to increased mind-body awareness. (Read on for more about your mind-body connection on page 14, and how dance cardio develops it.)

Exercise, and aerobic dance in particular, has been shown to help raise your self-esteem. Learning a new skill and boosting your health at the same time is bound to make you feel better about yourself!

What would you rather do: trudge on a treadmill for an hour or dance away the weight? Dancing is so fun that it doesn't even feel like exercise. That's why after a few minutes on the stationary bike you're ready to call it quits, but you're still pumped up after hours of shaking your groove thang at a club. If something is fun, you're more likely to do it — and more likely to drop pounds.

KNOW YOUR BODY

We'll be using the names of various muscles and body parts as we describe the cardio dance movements. If you are not sure what is what, check out the diagram on the following page to get in the know.

Muscular System

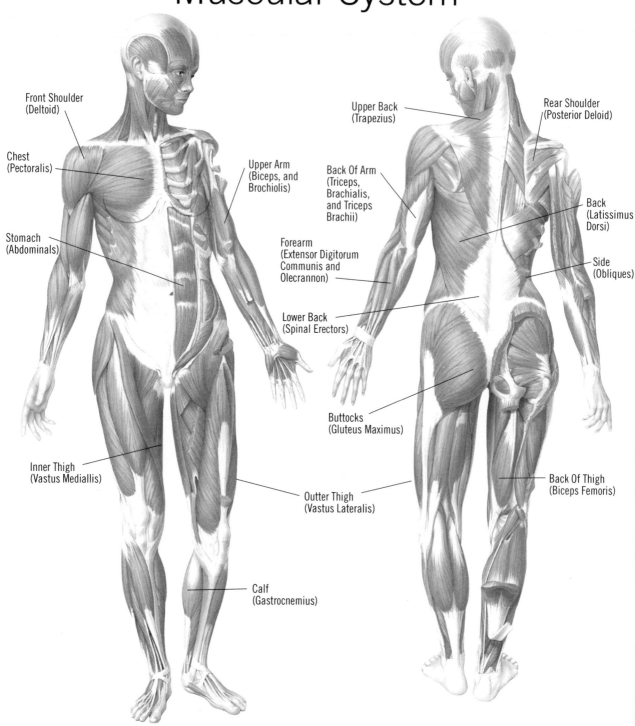

Front Shoulder
(Deltoid)

Chest
(Pectoralis)

Stomach
(Abdominals)

Upper Arm
(Biceps, and
Brochiolis)

Inner Thigh
(Vastus Mediallis)

Outter Thigh
(Vastus Lateralis)

Calf
(Gastrocnemius)

Upper Back
(Trapezius)

Rear Shoulder
(Posterior Deloid)

Back Of Arm
(Triceps,
Brachialis,
and Triceps
Brachii)

Back
(Latissimus
Dorsi)

Forearm
(Extensor Digitorum
Communis and
Olecrannon)

Side
(Obliques)

Lower Back
(Spinal Erectors)

Buttocks
(Gluteus Maximus)

Back Of Thigh
(Biceps Femoris)

BREATHING EASY

We do it every second of every day and rarely give it a thought. And yet, if we didn't do it, we wouldn't last for more than a few minutes. It's called breathing.

Since we have so much practice breathing, you'd think we'd be pretty good at it. But instead we tend to focus on the upper chest, taking short, shallow breaths. The result? Stress and anxiety may occur. And when we don't exhale all the air from our lungs, the gasses that remain turn into lactic acid in the muscles, which leads to soreness. Stress and soreness are not the way to get yourself excited about exercise!

Breathing deeply does more than ease stress and soreness — it may also benefit your heart. In a recent study, patients who learned to slow down their breathing through deep-breathing techniques actually ended up with higher levels of blood oxygen and performed better on exercise tests.

We want you be to able to dance until the proverbial cows come home — so let's learn how to breathe easy.

THORACIC BREATHING

In thoracic breathing, which is the type of breathing used in Pilates, you breathe into the middle lobes of your lungs so that the rib cage expands outward to the sides — which is why it's also known as "rib cage breathing." This breathing style gives you stamina as you exercise because it gets more oxygen to the muscles. To practice, lie on your back with four fingers

THORACIC BREATHING TIPS
- When doing cardio dance, inhale as you prepare for a move, and exhale as you execute it.
- Breathe in through the nose and out through the mouth.
- Breathe forcefully and completely.
- If you feel dizzy when you practice this type of breathing, try breathing less deeply.

of each hand lightly over your rib cage, with the fingers spread and pointing inward towards the center of your chest. Breathe so that you feel your hands moving out and away from one another. Once you get used to that, put one hand on your belly below the navel; your belly shouldn't rise as your rib cage expands.

DIAPHRAGMATIC BREATHING

We've all heard of deep breathing: books, articles, and yoga instructors all advise us to do it to relieve stress. The technical name for deep breathing is diaphragmatic breathing, because you are breathing from the diaphragm — the dome-shaped muscle that draws air into and out of the lungs — which means that as you breathe, your belly rises and falls. This is the type of breathing you'll do when you cool down after a cardio dance session. To practice diaphragmatic breathing, lie on your back with one hand on your rib cage and the other on your belly, as you did with the thoracic breathing exercise. However, this time as you breathe slowly in and out, you want your belly to rise and fall as you breathe, and your rib cage to remain still.

DEVELOP YOUR MIND-BODY CONNECTION

If you have ever exercised at your local gym, you've probably noticed two kinds of exercisers. One exerciser is reading a magazine and watching TV while she half-heartedly pedals the stationary bike or trudges on the treadmill. You may notice that this type of exerciser slouches, hangs onto the bar at the treadmill, and pedals hands-free on the stationary bike because she's reading holding a gossip magazine in front of her face.

The other exerciser may be plugged into her iPod, but she's clearly into what she's doing. Her posture is upright, and there's a look of

DEVELOPING YOUR MIND-BODY AWARENESS

Not sure how to get in touch with your inner you? Try these techniques for a sure-fire way to get your mind and body talking:

- Re-read how to practice thoracic and diaphragmatic breathing (see page 13 and opposite).
- When practicing, close your eyes and envision the path of how the air comes in through your nose, to your lungs and then travels on to the rest of your body as you are breathing out.
- As you are breathing out, engage your abdominal muscles so that they are slightly contracted (tense) yet still relaxed.
- Maintain that feeling of tension as you go into your next breath — this is the level of engagement and control you will focus on for each muscle as you move your inward focus from your abdominals to your legs.
- Repeat for each body part.

concentration on her face. She may be watching readouts that show her heart rate, distance covered, duration, and calories burned, adjusting her exercise intensity according to her body's response.

Which exerciser is getting the better workout? More than likely, it's the girl who is "plugged in" — she's not only plugged into her iPod, she's plugged in to her workout.

When you do any kind of exercise, be it bench presses or cardio dance, the secret to getting the most out of your workout is to develop a strong mind-body connection by focusing your thoughts on making your muscles move precisely the way you want them to (the practice of inward focus) — rather than just "going through the motions" and letting your mind wander during your exercise.

By paying greater attention (with your mind) to what is being experienced by your muscles and breath (within your body), you will find that you experience a heightened level of satisfaction and enjoyment with your cardio dance workout. Developing your mind-body awareness doesn't just bring satisfaction to your workout; it also helps to prevent unwanted injuries that may occur from getting your steps backwards or turning the wrong way during a combination. And as an added bonus, recent scientific evidence suggests that a strong mind-body connection can also help you lose weight.

As you start paying attention — really paying attention — to your exercise, you'll learn to enjoy the rhythm of the music, the feel of the moves, and the natural way your body responds to ELLE's fun cardio dance workout!

Now that we've covered the basics with you, you are ready to go on to Chapter 2, Getting Started, where we'll cover the technical details of your workout, from what to wear during your exercise session, to where to workout, to how to assess your fitness level.

Remember, the ELLE Glam Fitness Complete Cardio workout is all about dancing in the moment. As you perform your cardio dance routine, try not to think about what you had for breakfast or the work that's waiting for you once you finish. Instead, think about what you're doing:

How precise can you be in your movements? How do the movements feel? How does your body feel — are you exhilarated, tired, do you feel any discomfort? (Another benefit to dancing in the moment is that you'll recognize any problems, such as a move that's causing you pain, and be able to make corrections.) With time and practice, you will become more fluid and the movements will no longer seem like work; instead you will find yourself dancing just to dance, rather than to exercise.

Are you ready? Read on!

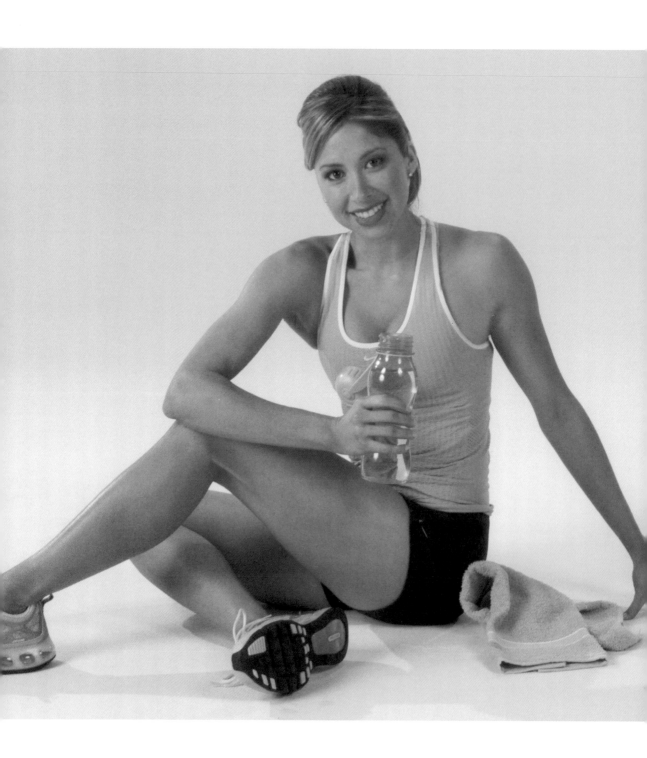

CHAPTER 2
GETTING STARTED

Now that you've got the low-down on how to effectively ho-down, we'll put you in the know so you can get started with your ELLE Glam Fitness Complete Cardio workout. We'll help you determine your exercise goals, find the perfect place to practice, and even share why, though it may seem appealing at the time, wearing your favorite pair of old sweats isn't always the best idea.

PLAN TO SUCCEED

For most, the hardest part of exercising is simply getting started. While many are well intended ("I'll start Monday," or "I'll do it tomorrow"), tomorrow comes and goes while they find themselves reiterating the same words over again.

The ones who do succeed at getting started are the ones who have taken the time to lay out a plan. It's easy to say that you are going to do your ELLE Glam Fitness Complete Cardio workout every day for 365 days. However, as you are soon to discover, saying that you are going to do it versus actually doing it are two different matters entirely. That's where having a rock solid exercise plan comes in.

Read on to develop your sure-fire strategy to getting more fit, the ELLE Glam Fitness way.

STEP 1: SET A GOAL

Exercising without a goal is like getting in your car without knowing where you want to drive. A goal gives you a sense of purpose — something to work towards, and something to measure your progress against. Successful goal setting is S.M.A.R.T.:

S FOR SPECIFIC: What exactly do you hope to achieve? Instead of saying you want to exercise, say that you want to do the ELLE Glam Fitness Complete Cardio workout twice a week. Instead of saying you want to "lose some flab," choose an amount you want to lose.

M FOR MOTIVATING: You need to be excited about what you want to achieve! If the idea of losing weight makes you want to snooze, perhaps it's not the right goal for you at this moment. Maybe boosting your overall health, building your strength, increasing your flexibility or lowering your cholesterol levels are more motivating for you.

A FOR ACHIEVABLE: Nothing is more of a buzz kill than a goal too difficult to achieve. No one can (safely) lose 60 pounds in two months. Give yourself a break!

R FOR RELEVANT: The goal needs to make sense for you. If you choose some pie-in-the-sky goal because it looks good on paper — like "My goal is to work out for an hour every day, rain or shine, in sickness or in health" — chances are you'll ditch it within the week. Create a goal that works with your schedule and abilities.

T FOR TRACKABLE: If you can't track your goal, how will you know when you've achieved it? We're talking numbers here: Instead of setting a goal to lose some random amount of weight in some random amount of time, resolve to lose X pounds by Y date.

STEP 2: WRITE YOUR GOAL DOWN

Experts state that an unwritten goal is merely wishful thinking. By writing your goal down, you commit to yourself that your goal is important enough to work towards and achieve. Turn to page 122 to record your goal — it will come in handy later as you go through the following steps.

Goals that are achievable are goals that are realistic! For example, a goal of losing 20 pounds in a week is NOT realistic. A more realistic and attainable goal would be listed as "lose 20 pounds: 1 pound a week for 20 weeks".

STEP 3: DO YOUR HOMEWORK

Now that you've identified your goal, you want to jump right into working on it, right? If you can, hold off until you've done your homework. Make sure you completely understand what you need to do for yourself — poor planning or no planning at all can easily curtail your efforts. It's frustrating to be working your tail off to not see any progress. A solid "how to" plan can help you work smarter, not harder! Talk with those in the know around you — people who have already achieved what you are looking to do for yourself. Find out what you are going to need in terms of time, energy, and effort to achieve your goals. You might want to consider hiring a professional who can help you develop your plan of attack and can provide a great source of support when the going gets a little tough!

STEP 4: SET A TIME FRAME

A goal without a set beginning and end is a goal that can be easily put off. Once you understand what is involved, you should be able to realistically plan how long it will take you to get there, and make all necessary adjustments to your schedule to accommodate the time required to achieve your goal. Recording your start date and end date will provide you with the vital ingredient for achieving your goal. You'll find that we've provided a goals worksheet on page 22 to help get you started.

STEP 5: SET BENCHMARKS

This is the easy part! You've done your homework and set your time frame. Now, working backwards from your completion date and end goal, break up your main goal into smaller sub-goals that each carry its own time frame and benchmark within your main goal.
For example, if your goal is to lose 20 pounds in 20 weeks at 1 pound a week, break those 20 weeks up into five 4-week periods. Your first benchmark would be at week 4 with a goal of losing 4 pounds. Your second benchmark would be at week 8, with a goal of losing 8 pounds total since you started, etc. Remember, it is important to have tangible, measurable goals; if you can't measure your progress, it is very difficult to not know how you are progressing. Also, measurable results allow you to see if your current formula is working for you. If you aren't making the progress you planned, then you can fix your formula early on, without wasting a lot of energy on something that isn't working! !

STEP 6: PLAN ONE STEP AT A TIME

Nothing is more frustrating than not getting to your goal because you have planned to do too much, too soon. A successful exercise program needs to be broken down into manageable steps. For example, if you want to start exercising but haven't worked out before, planning to exercise 5 times a week from the get-go is not the best place to start. A more realistic and attainable start (see S.M.A.R.T. goal setting earlier in this chapter) would be exercising once a week. Why? It will give your body time to safely adapt to the physiological stress of exercise and prevent the I-am-so-sore-I-can-hardly-walk-let-alone-exercise-again feeling that comes from overdoing it. Example: The S.M.A.R.T. strategy for getting started would be:

Start exercising 1 time a week for 3 weeks. Once you are easily able to complete all 3 exercise sessions in the course of the 3 weeks, then move on to exercising 2 times per week for the next 4 weeks. Once again, if you are easily able to complete all sessions in the course of the 4 weeks, then move on to exercising 3 times per week for the next 5 weeks.

GLAM GOAL SETTER

JUST DO IT. There will be times when you are unable to exercise for a week or two, possibly even longer. Don't feel guilty or disappointed in yourself, just start your routine again as quickly as you can.

PLAN YOUR WORKOUTS. In Chapter 7 we've included some additional routines to try once you are up to the challenge. Make photocopies of them, and put them in your dayplanner on the days that you are planning to do each particular routine. Once you have done the entire routine, cross each move off your copy. Make notes and changes for your next workout based on your previous performance.

TRACK YOUR PROGRESS. Use the weight-loss and body-composition sheet (page 159) to help you determine your progress. Having a consistent record of your body weight and girth measurements can help you better determine how well your fitness plan is working for you.

STEP 7: MAKE YOUR PLAN LIVABLE AND DOABLE

In the first few weeks of your new exercise program, you may find that you'll have a few false starts before you succeed at making the ELLE Glam Cardio Dance program a regular, consistent part of your fitness lifestyle. But don't despair, the good news is there is no one right way to get in shape, so if you can only do 1 time versus the 5 you were planning on, you'll still come out ahead of the game.

STEP 8: BE ACCOUNTABLE

Accountability is the only way to be successful in your endeavor to achieving your goal. Being honest with yourself about your strengths and weaknesses will lead you to have greater understanding of what works for you in your life, and what you are capable of achieving. Record what works and what doesn't work for you as you proceed through your journey. When the going gets rough, look back to see what was different for you when things where working well. Having this type of insight will help you to overcome obstacles along the way.

STEP 9: GIVE YOURSELF PERMISSION

No matter what, the journey to achieving your goal will not be 100% what you want it to be. You won't always be able to make your workout session, or you may not always have the correct food available to you. Remember, your success lies in your consistency to be able to enact your plan over the long haul, not just today. If today wasn't perfect, don't sweat it, you always have tomorrow. Making the best decision for you based on what is available to you is the trick to becoming successful in achieving your goal. If you have a bad day, you haven't blown it. Pick yourself up and get back on track. It's okay! It is very difficult to be 100% on plan all the time, even with the best preparation and planning.

STEP 10: PUT YOUR GAME FACE ON

The success of your efforts lay in not only how well you plan out your goal, but what your mindset is during the process as well. Negative mindsets lead to unsuccessful effort, which, in turn, ultimately leads to failure and the "I'm never going to get there" feeling.

Reaching your goal is a journey, one that is not always easy. Having the right mindset coupled with a realistic plan will teach you a lot about what you are truly capable of achieving along the way. You'll find that you'll be able to overcome obstacles (such as how you are going to continue your exercise program when you travel for work), objectively troubleshoot sticking points (like how to get yourself back in the groove of working out after you have missed a few workout sessions) and see yourself in a different light (you'll feel good knowing that you are taking control of your fitness, even though you may not exactly be where you want to be yet) to effectively make the ELLE Glam Fitness Cardio Dance Workout a healthy lifestyle tool that you will continue to use as you settle into your new fitness routine.

Now you've identified your goal and made sure it is S.M.A.R.T., you are just about to start rearranging your living room furniture to test drive the ELLE Glam Fitness Complete Cardio workout in the next chapter. But don't turn the page yet! There are a few more things left to do before you can safely start exercising.

VISIT YOUR MD

Yes, we know you're a young, glam female — but we also know that visiting your doctor before beginning a new exercise program has many benefits that can make your workouts more effective. A routine check-up will tell you your baseline blood pressure, weight and cholesterol readings, which will provide a starting point that you can measure against when you visit your doctor in a year's time. A check-up can also provide you with instant goals: high blood pressure? Your new goal is to lower your blood pressure. Ten pounds overweight? Now you know how much you need to lose. That said, grab a pen and answer the following questions. The results will let you know if it's safe to start exercising before seeing your doc.

CHECK UP: ARE YOU READY TO EXERCISE?

Answer the following questions **YES** or **NO**.

1 Has your doctor ever told you that you have a heart condition and that you should only do activity recommended by an M.D.?
2 Do you feel pain in your chest when you're physically active?
3 In the past month, have you had chest pain when you were not doing physical activity?
4 Do you ever lose your balance because of dizziness, or do you ever lose consciousness?
5 Do you have a bone or joint problem that could be made worse by a change in your physical activity level?
6 Is your doctor currently prescribing drugs (for example, water pills) for your blood pressure or a heart condition?
7 Do you know of any other reason why you should not exercise?*

If you answered **YES** to one or more questions, call your doctor and discuss your exercise plans. Tell him that you have taken a PAR-Q (Physical Activity Readiness Questionnaire) and which questions you answered yes to. Depending on your answers, you doctor may advise you to start exercising slowly and build up gradually. Or, you may need to restrict your exercise until you have had a complete physical and obtain clearance from your doctor.

If you honestly answered **NO** to all of the questions, you can start exercising! However, begin slowly and build up gradually.

* Adapted from the Canadian Society for Exercise Physiology, Inc., 1994

HOW FIT ARE YOU?

Another good thing to do before starting your ELLE Glam Fitness workout is determine exactly how fit you are. Don't worry, we are not going to ask you to run until you drop or do a pushup test, but the following quick fitness assessment will help to give you a better understanding of how hard you should be working during your exercise session.

USING RATE OF PERCEIVED EXERTION TO RATE YOUR FITNESS LEVEL

The Rate of Perceived Exertion (RPE) is how hard you feel like your body is working. It is based on the physical sensations a person experiences during physical activity, including increased heart rate, increased respiration or breathing rate, increased sweating, and muscle fatigue. Although this is a subjective measure, a person's exertion rating may provide a fairly good estimate of the actual heart rate during physical activity. For our purposes, we are going to be using RPE to give you a more concrete way to identify the level of intensity (difficulty) of your workout. While you are exercising, you rate how difficult a movement feels to perform using a scale of 1 to 10. A rating of 1 means that the movement is very, very, easy to perform (requiring no effort at all), whereas a rating of 10 is the absolute hardest to perform, requiring maximal effort (you can't work any harder).

Using the chart on the following page, rate each of the below exercises. Total up your points and match them with the Fitness Level Chart results, below, to see where your fitness level is, and at what intensity you should start your cardio dance workout:

- climbing 2 flights of stairs;

- carrying a full laundry basket up 1 flight of stairs;

- walking at a moderate pace for 20 minutes without stopping;

- jogging for 10 minutes without stopping;

- running for 10 minutes without stopping.

FITNESS LEVEL CHART

Score 1–10 points   Advanced Exerciser

Score 20–35 points   Intermediate Exerciser

Score 36–50 points   Beginning Exerciser

RPE SCALE	FEELS LIKE	EXERCISE LEVEL	AMOUNT OF EFFORT	TALK TEST
1	sitting down and reading	not hard at all	no effort required	can carry full conversations
2	sitting down carrying on a light conversation	very easy	requires almost no effort	can carry on full conversations
3	talking steadily on the phone while walking around	easy	only requires a little bit of effort	can carry full conversations
4	conversing while carrying grocery bags	less easy	requires some effort	can carry shorter conversations
5	conversing while climbing stairs	moderate	requires effort	can carry short conversations
6	conversing while climbing stairs holding grocery bags	challenging	requires more effort	can speak in short sentences
7	conversing while taking stairs two at a time	more challenging	requires most effort	can speak short phrases
8	conversing while taking two stairs at a time holding grocery bags	very challenging	requires all effort	speaking is difficult
9	conversing while running two stairs at a time	exceptionnally challenging	requires maximum effort	can speak a few words
10	conversing while running two stairs at a time holding grocery bags	maximally challenging	requires full-out effort	can't speak at all

HOW DID YOU SCORE?

If you're a Beginning Exerciser, you'll start off at a lower intensity level to allow your body to become used to consistent exercise; if you're an Intermediate or Advanced Exerciser, your body is ready to work slightly harder during your exercise sessions.

If you are a Beginning Exerciser, a good place to start on the RPE scale is a 4 or 5. As you become more comfortable with your workout and it becomes easier to do, raise your intensity to a 5 or 6 by speeding up the music you workout to, or add additional dance combinations into your routine. The higher the intensity of your workout, the harder you work, which means the more calories you'll burn.

If you are an Intermediate/Advanced Exerciser, start your workouts at a level 6 or 7. After you are fully warm, raise the intensity to an 8 or 9 for a minute or two, and then bring it back down to the 6 or 7 you started at. This type of training is called interval training, and is most effective for burning calories without burning you out by exercising at too high of a level. In the chart, we've outlined some sample scenarios to help you determine the right intensity level to start at and how hard to push yourself during your following workouts. You'll notice in our chart there is a column titled "Talk Test." We've included that as an even easier way to tell how hard you are working. The Talk Test has been proven as the simplest method to determine the appropriate exercise intensity. Here's how it works: When you can no longer speak full sentences comfortably, you are most likely exercising at the right intensity. However, when speech becomes difficult, you are working too hard and need to slow your pace down.

Make a copy of the chart and keep it with your workout logs to refer to until you know exactly how hard you are working!

WHAT TO WEAR

Don't be tempted to dance in your jammies, your jeans, or those old sweats you wear on your "fat days." Changing into clothes that you chose specifically for exercise puts you into the right mindset to get moving. In fact, many regular exercisers say that even if they don't feel like training, they put on their workout clothes — and this makes them want to exercise. Exercise clothes are also more comfortable to move in than tight pants, and they make you feel sexier than your "fat sweats," which will keep your motivation up as you exercise.

DANCE FLOOR FASHION

The best workout clothes are loose enough to move freely in, but not so loose that you end up tripping over your bell bottoms. Think yoga clothes: form-fitting, stretchy pants and a fitted tank or T. Plain cotton is fine, but if it's hot where you live you may want to check out exercise clothes made from breathable materials that wick moisture from the skin, such as Under Armour brand clothing.

BEATING BOUNCE

The skin and much of the tissue in your breasts is elastic. Researchers have determined that 36C breasts can bounce as much as 4.7 inches up and down when their owner runs at 5.6 mph. In other words: Ouch. So find a sports bra that minimizes bouncing — if you have to jump up and down to figure this out, do it in the changing room.
The first sports bra was made from two jockstraps sewn together, now you can find sports bras that camouflage and protect nipples, and even have a mesh fabric that lets the skin breathe.

A SHOE-IN

Finally, you'll need a good pair of aerobic shoes or cross trainers. Don't wear your old running shoes, as these don't have enough bounce or ankle support for cardio dance. In fact, don't wear your old aerobic shoes, either; you should replace your workout shoes every 6 to 12 months.

MUSIC TO GROOVE TO

You can choose any kind of music that makes you want to move — as long as it's not so fast that you can't keep up with the beat. If you have no clue where to start, check out WorkOutMusic.com and AerobicsMusic.com for CDs with names like Tribal Beat Workout 1 and Top 40 Hip Hop Party 3.

PICK A PLACE

You can do your ELLE Glam Dance Cardio Workout anywhere.
Well, not anywhere but you can dance inside or outside.
If you decide to dance indoors, choose an area with a hard floor or a dense carpet. Avoid area rugs or loose-pile carpets, which can make you lose your balance. If you'd rather dance outdoors, look for an area with short grass or packed dirt instead of concrete, which has no give.

A FINAL WORD

The best way to practice your dance moves is often. Don't worry about being perfect. Don't even worry about being particularly good. The goal is to get moving, have fun, and burn calories.

In the next chapter we will get you warmed up and ready to groove!

ELLE

GLAM FITNESS
COMPLETE CARDIO

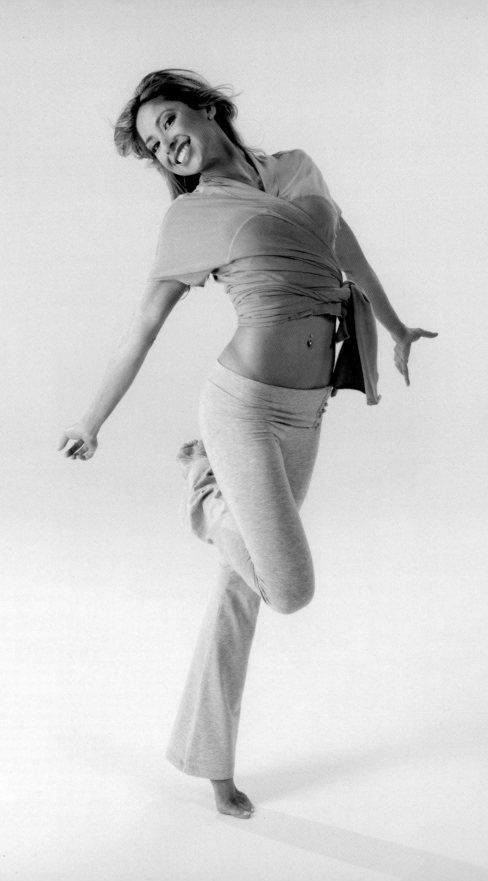

CHAPTER 3
THE WARM-UP ROUTINE

The warm-up is the most important part of the workout, but most often, it is also the part that is most overlooked. It's easy to overlook it — you'll be warm anyway once you exercise, right? So why waste the time warming up?

Warming up properly ensures that you prepare your body in a safe way for the more intense work that is to come later — the gradual build of a good warm-up allows your body adequate time to raise your heart rate, respiration and core temperature to the proper level so you can perform your ELLE Glam Fitness Complete Cardio dance routine safely and effectively, with less chance of injury.

On the following pages you'll find a fun warm-up routine that gets your heart going and your body warm. After you are warm, we'll take a moment to stretch and then move into some beginning dance combinations.

The following pages describe each movement in detail, so that you can take it one step at a time. We encourage you to use this chapter page-by-page for your first few workouts, as we've included the number of steps you should be doing for each movement, so you can keep exercising as you learn. At the end of each section is the full routine for you to try. When you become more comfortable with the warm-up routine and no longer need the visual clues, turn to Chapter 7 for more advanced routines.

Never stretch cold: You actually increase your risk of injury. Always be sure that you have performed some light movements and elevated your heart rate slightly so that your body is warm before doing any stretching.

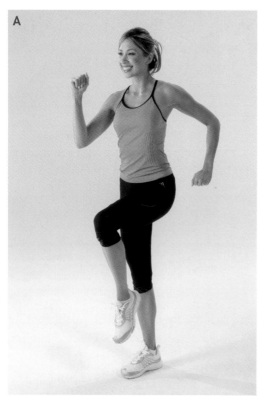

WARM-UP EXERCISES

MARCH
(16 steps in place)

START POSITION: Stand with your feet hip-width apart, arms at your sides.

MOVEMENT:

A) Keeping your head up and abdominals tight, raise your left leg by lifting your knee to hip height. Gently bring your right arm forward to eye level in a "swinging" motion, with your elbow softly bent at 90 degrees.

B) Return your left leg to the floor and repeat on the other side, being sure to alternate the arm motion as you raise the opposite leg.

MARCH OUT WIDE
(8 steps out to each side)

Once you have mastered the March, this variation is easy to implement.

Keeping your head up and abdominals tight, raise your left leg by lifting your knee to hip height. Gently bring your right arm forward to eye level in a "swinging" motion, with your elbow softly bent at 90 degrees.

As you return your left leg to the floor, place it hip-width to the side of you, outside of your normal marching stance. Repeat on the other side, being sure to alternate the arm motion as you raise the opposite leg.

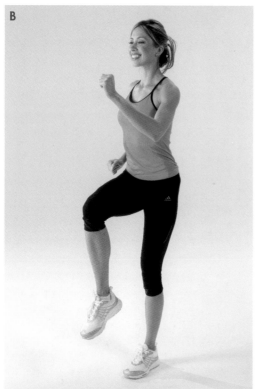

STEP TOUCH SIDE TO SIDE

(alternate 8 step touches to the right with 8 step touches to the left)

START POSITION: A) Stand with your feet close together, arms at your sides.

MOVEMENT:

B) Looking straight ahead, step out to your right side with your right leg. Keep your arms relaxed with your elbows softly bent at 90 degrees.

C) Stepping onto your right leg, complete the movement by bringing your left leg to your right leg, "touching" the floor next to your right foot with the ball of your left foot. Repeat back to the other side.

A
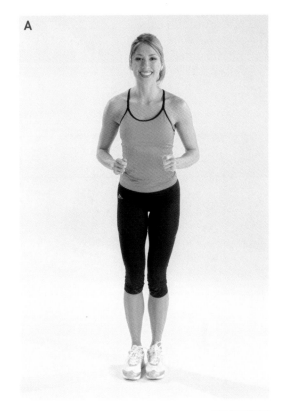

B
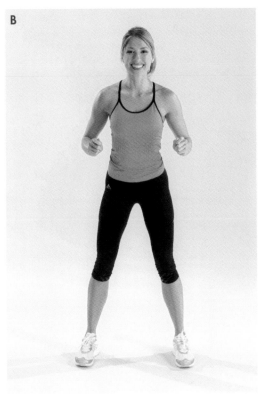

C
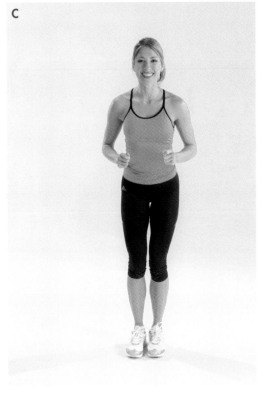

TRAVEL UP AND BACK
(16 steps in place)

START POSITION: Stand with your feet close together, arms at your sides.

MOVEMENT:

A) With your right leg, step forward and slightly out to the side, at a 45-degree angle in front of you.

B) Following the same motion that you set with your right leg, bring your left leg forward to where your right leg is so that now both feet are together.

C) Continuing the forward motion, step your left leg out and slightly to the side, ensuring that your hips are still facing in front of you. Complete the motion by bringing your right leg up to meet your left leg.

After you have traveled forward for a few steps, repeat the process by traveling backwards until you reach your original starting point.

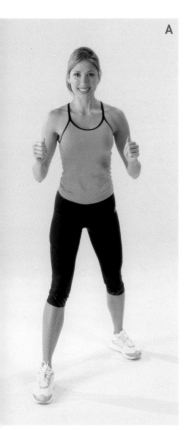
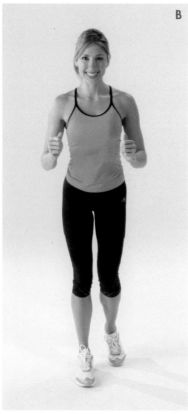
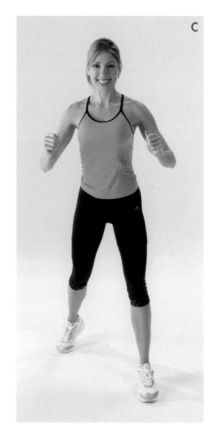

THE ROUTINE

16 steps in place = **MARCH**

8 steps out to the side = **MARCH OUT WIDE**

8 steps in place = **MARCH**

8 steps side to side = **STEP TOUCH SIDE TO SIDE**

4 steps forward = **TRAVEL UP**

4 steps back = **TRAVEL BACK**

8 steps side to side = **STEP TOUCH SIDE TO SIDE**

4 steps forward = **TRAVEL UP**

4 steps back = **TRAVEL BACK**

8 steps side to side = **STEP TOUCH SIDE TO SIDE**

8 steps side to side = **STEP TOUCH SIDE TO SIDE** (Low)*

8 steps side to side = **STEP TOUCH SIDE TO SIDE**

4 steps forward = **TRAVEL UP**

4 steps back = **TRAVEL BACK** (Low)

4 steps forward = **TRAVEL UP**

4 steps back = **TRAVEL BACK** (Low)

4 steps forward = **TRAVEL UP**

4 steps back = **TRAVEL BACK** (Low)

8 steps side to side = **STEP TOUCH**

8 steps in place = **MARCH**

8 steps out to the side = **MARCH OUT WIDE**

* This is an advanced movement. Bend at the hips so that your torso is at a 45-degree angle and your chest is slightly towards the floor. Maintain this position for the entire combination.

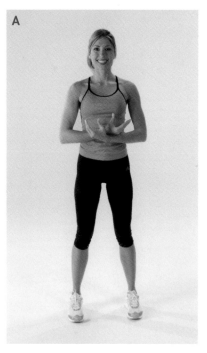

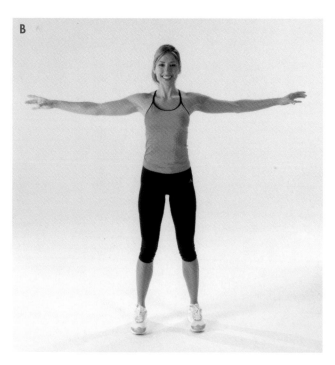

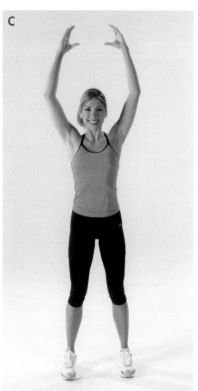

STRETCHES

ARMS UP STRETCH *(2 times)*

START POSITION: A) Stand with your feet shoulder-width apart, crossing your hands in front of your rib cage.

MOVEMENT:

B) Keeping your legs in place, make the motion of a circle by bringing your hands down towards the floor and up towards the ceiling, keeping each arm out to the side.

C) Finish making the circle by bringing your hands above your head.

Return your hands to their start position and repeat.

Don't forget to breathe! Breathing in when it is easiest and out when it is hardest ensures you have enough oxygen to make it through your full workout!

LOOK SIDE TO SIDE
(4 times each side)

START POSITION: Stand with your feet shoulder-width apart, arms relaxed at your sides.

MOVEMENT:

A) Staying in place, turn only your head to the right, keeping the rest of your body facing forward. Be sure to only turn your head as far as it is comfortable for you.

B) Complete the movement by doing the same to the left side.

A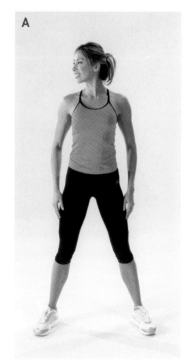
B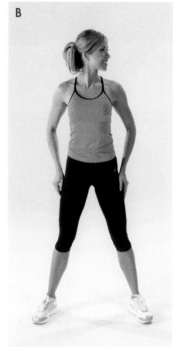

CHIN DOWN
(4 times down, 4 times up)

START POSITION: Stand with your feet shoulder-width apart, arms relaxed at your sides.

MOVEMENT:

A) Keeping your body relaxed, bring your chin towards your chest so that you are looking at the floor.

B) Reverse the movement, returning your chin back to the original upright position.

A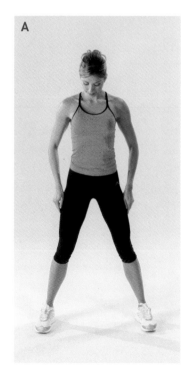
B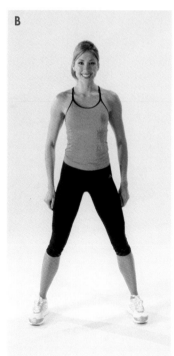

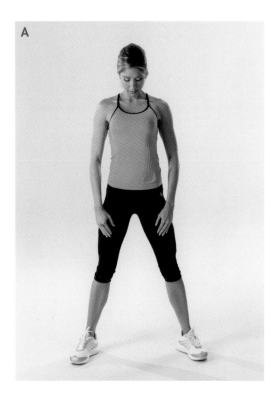

CIRCLE NECK ROLLS
(4 rolls each side)

START POSITION: A) Stand with your feet shoulder-width apart, arms relaxed at your sides. Your chin should be towards your chest, eyes towards the floor.

MOVEMENT:

B) Slowly roll your head towards your right shoulder, stopping when your ear is in line with your shoulder.

C) Reverse the movement so that you roll your head back down and up to your left side.

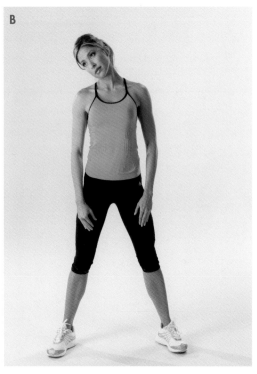

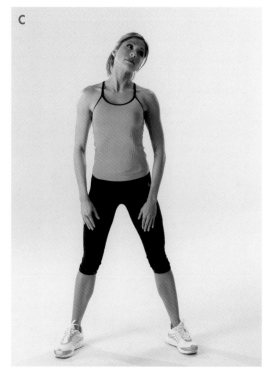

FLAT BACK DOWN
(3 down, 2 up)

START POSITION: A) Stand with your feet shoulder-width apart and your knees slightly bent. Lean forward 90 degrees at your hips, supporting your upper body by placing your hands on your thighs.

MOVEMENT:

B) In a slow, controlled fashion, round out your shoulder blades by dropping your chin to your chest and pulling your navel in as you lift your torso towards the ceiling.

C) Slowly roll up into a full upright position.

D) Reverse the movement by gently arching your back as you descend into the original start position. Repeat.

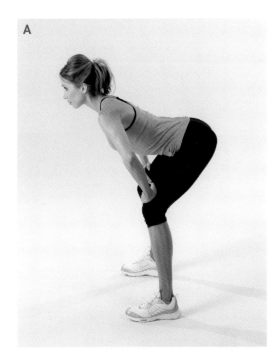

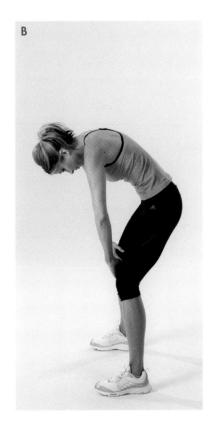

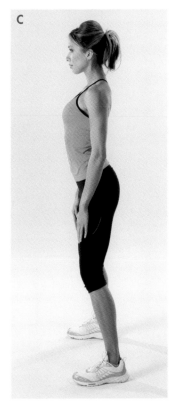

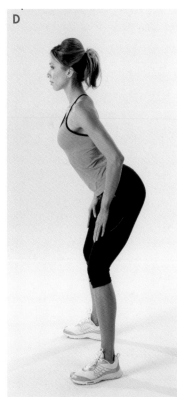

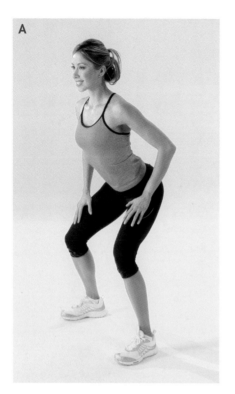

SINGLE ROUND BACK AND UP
(6 single backs in place)

START POSITION: A) Stand with your feet shoulder-width apart and your knees slightly bent. Lean forward 90 degrees at your hips, supporting your upper body by placing your hands on your thighs. Keep your chest up so there is a slight arch in your back.

MOVEMENT:

B) In a slow controlled fashion, round out your shoulder blades by dropping your chin to your chest and pulling your navel in. Do not roll all the way up to an upright position; instead, return directly to your start position from here.

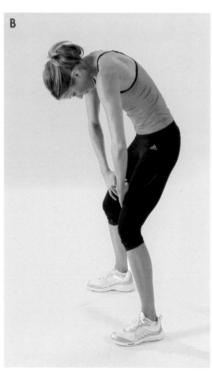

RAG DOLL STRETCH
(1 ful body stretch)

START POSITION: A) Standing with your feet wide, lean all the way forward so that your hands are relaxed on the floor and you are looking through your legs.

MOVEMENT:

B) Lifting from your shoulder blades, slowly roll your torso upright in a relaxed manner.

C) Once you are upright, finish the movement by rolling your shoulders back.

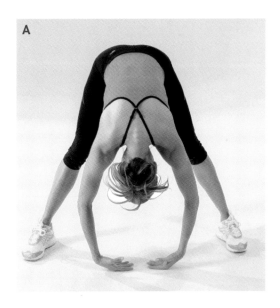

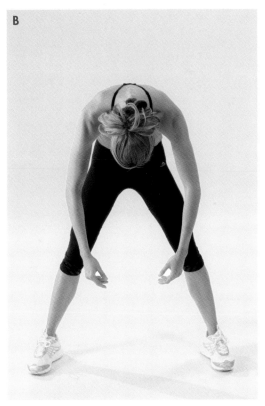

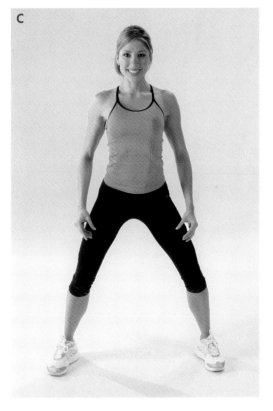

THE ROUTINE SO FAR

WARM-UP

16 steps in place = MARCH

8 steps out to the side = MARCH OUT WIDE

8 steps in place = MARCH

8 steps side to side = STEP TOUCH SIDE TO SIDE

4 steps forward = TRAVEL UP

4 steps back = TRAVEL BACK

8 steps side to side = STEP TOUCH SIDE TO SIDE

4 steps forward = TRAVEL UP

4 steps back = TRAVEL BACK

8 steps side to side = STEP TOUCH SIDE TO SIDE

8 steps side to side = STEP TOUCH SIDE TO SIDE (Low)

8 steps side to side = STEP TOUCH SIDE TO SIDE

4 steps forward = TRAVEL UP

4 steps back = TRAVEL BACK (Low)

4 steps forward = TRAVEL UP

4 steps back = TRAVEL BACK (Low)

4 steps forward = TRAVEL UP

4 steps back = TRAVEL BACK (Low)

8 steps side to side = STEP TOUCH

8 steps in place = MARCH

8 steps out to the side = MARCH OUT WIDE

STRETCH

2 arm circles = ARMS UP STRETCH

4 looks to the right, 4 looks to the left = LOOK SIDE TO SIDE

4 chin down, 4 chin up = CHIN DOWN

4 CIRCLE NECK ROLLS

1 arm circle = ARMS UP

3 flat back down, 2 round back up = FLAT BACK DOWN

6 single back staying down = SINGLE BACK

1 full body roll up = RAG DOLL STRETCH

1 arm circle = ARMS UP STRETCH

ISOLATION SEQUENCES

SHOULDER SIDE TO SIDE

(4 to each side)

START POSITION: A) Stand with your feet wide apart, arms relaxed at your sides.

MOVEMENT:

B) Bringing your left shoulder forward and right shoulder back, lean to your left side, slightly bending your knees.

C) Keeping your knees bent, bring your weight over to your right side by dipping your body down, then up, as you raise your left shoulder to your right side. Reverse the motion to repeat.

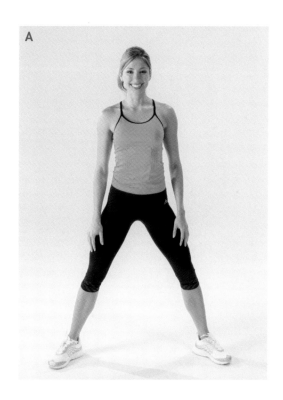

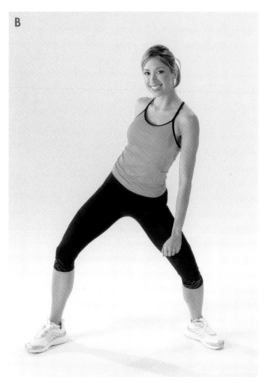

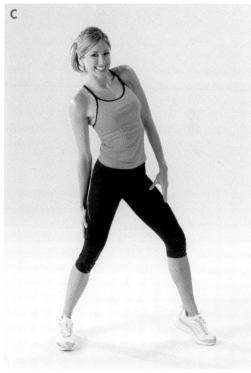

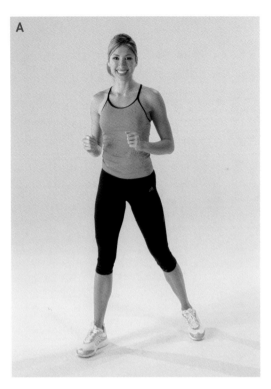

GRAPEVINE

(step, crossover, step, touch: 4 times to the right, 4 times to the left)

START POSITION: A) Stand with your feet shoulder-width apart, arms softly bent at the elbows.

MOVEMENT:

B) Cross your left foot over your right foot, traveling to the side. Bring your back leg (right leg) out and to the side.

C) Bring your left leg in to meet you right leg, "touching" the floor next to it. Reverse and repeat.

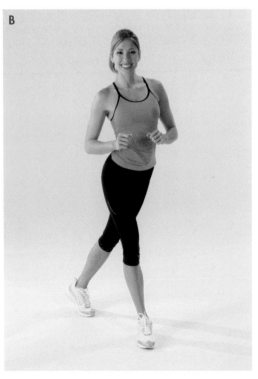

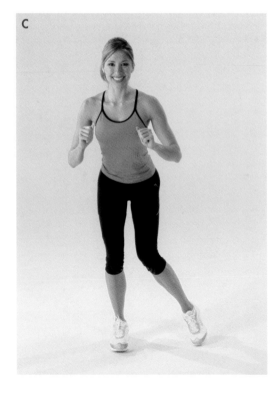

PLIE
(4 plies)

START POSITION: A) Stand with your feet wide apart, crossing your hands in front of your rib cage.

MOVEMENT:

B) Gently bending your legs as you raise your arms, make the motion of a circle by bringing your hands down towards the floor and up towards the ceiling.

Complete the movement by straightening your legs as you return your hands to their original position.

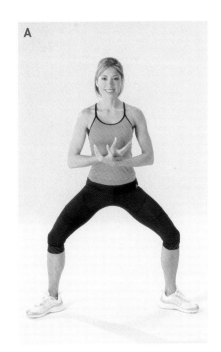
A

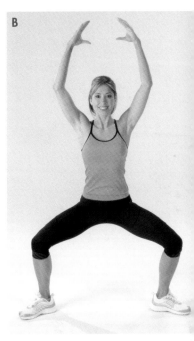
B

PLIE WITH ARMS TO THE FRONT
(4 plies)

START POSITION: A) Stand with your feet wide apart, arms straight out in front of you at chest level.

MOVEMENT:

B) Gently bending your legs as you move your arms, make the motion of a half circle by bringing your hands out to your sides.

Complete the movement by straightening your legs as you return your hands to their original position.

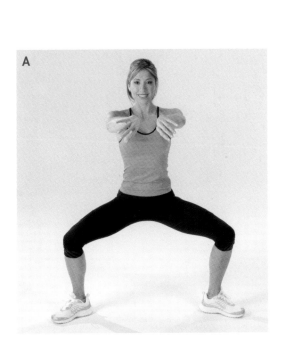
A

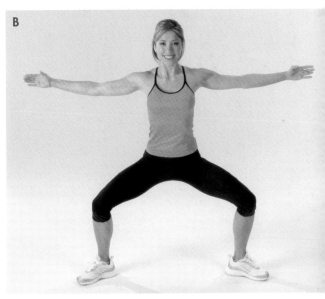
B

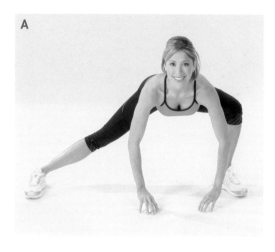

HAMSTRING STRETCH
(2 stretches to each side)

START POSITION: Stand with your feet wide apart, arms relaxed at your sides.

MOVEMENT:

A) Leaning forward, bend at the hips so that your fingertips can touch the floor. Keeping your head up and eyes ahead, lean to your left side by bending your left knee to 90 degrees. Keep your right leg straight.

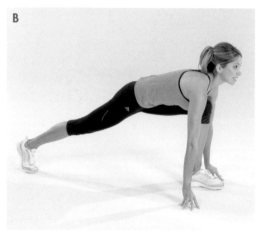

B) Walk your fingertips around your left leg, so that your torso now rests on your thigh and your arms straddle each side of your left leg.

C) Advanced finish: Keeping your hands in place, straighten your legs so that your torso is parallel to the ground. Slowly return to upright and repeat.

D) Beginner variation: Keeping your torso at a 45-degree angle, place your hands on your left thigh, gently bending your back leg until you feel a stretch. Reverse and repeat on the other side.

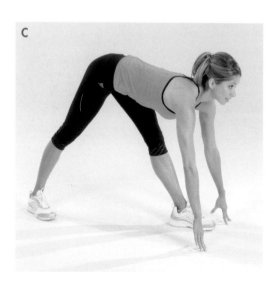

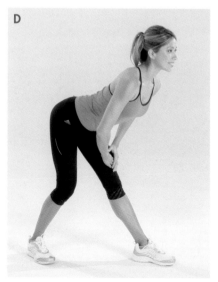

WIDE LEG STRETCH
(2 stretches)

START POSITION: Stand with your feet shoulder width apart, arms relaxed at your sides.

MOVEMENT:

A) Staying in place, raise your arms out to your sides.

B) Bringing your arms up overhead, bend forward at the waist until the palms of your hands are flat on the floor. Slowly return to upright and repeat.

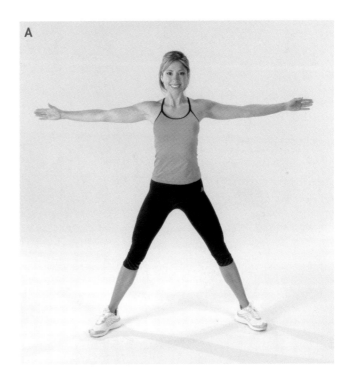

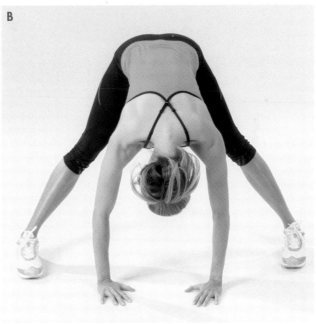

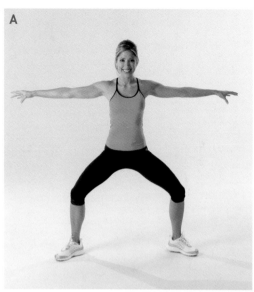

PIVOT STRETCH

(2 pivots to the right, 2 pivots to the left)

START POSITION: A) Stand with your feet wide apart, arms out to the sides, palms down and knees slightly bent.

MOVEMENT:

B) Leaving your right arm in place, slowly bring your left arm over to meet your right arm by turning your torso and hips towards your right side. Drop your left knee towards the floor.

C) Complete the movement by meeting your left arm to your right arm. Reverse the motion and repeat on the other side.

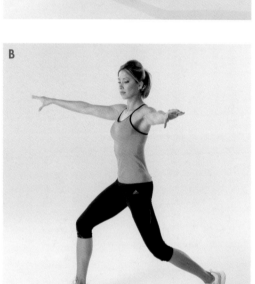

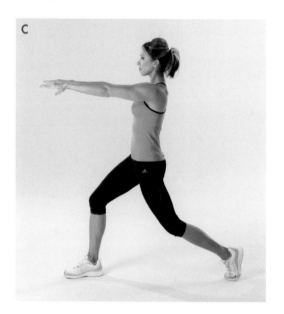

SHAKE AND SHIMEE
(4 shakes to the right, 4 shimees to the left)

START POSITION: Stand with your feet shoulder width apart, arms relaxed at your sides.

MOVEMENT:

A) Bringing your arms overhead, shift your weight to the right side, quickly pushing your left hip forward at the same time.

B) Quickly reverse the movement and do the same as you shift your weight over to your left side.

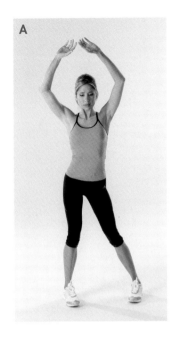
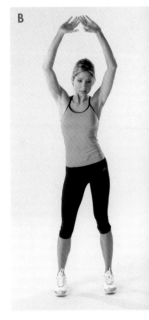

SIDE TO SIDE STRETCH
(4 to the right, 4 to the left)

START POSITION: A) Stand with your feet wide apart, arms out to your sides, palms down and knees slightly bent.

MOVEMENT:

B) Staying in place, lean your torso to the right, keeping your arm straight as you extend it out to the side. Rotate your palm up as you do so.

C) Reverse and repeat as you move towards the left side.

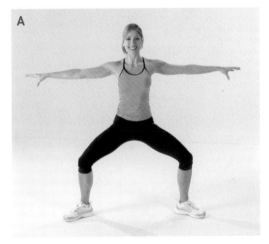

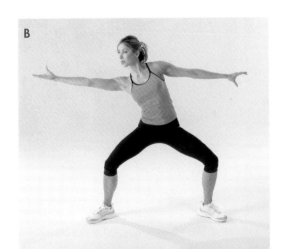
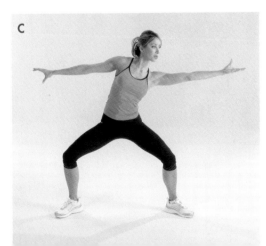

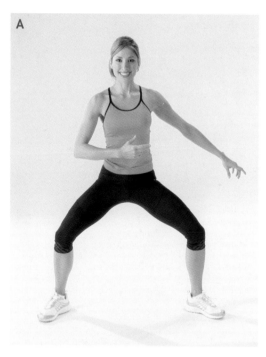

SHOULDER ROLL
(4 rolls to the right, 4 rolls to the left)

START POSITION: A) Stand with your feet wide apart, left arm out to the side, right arm softly bent in front of your rib cage.

MOVEMENT:

B) Shift your weight to the right side of your body by bending your right knee and dipping your hip down and out to the side. At the same time, roll your right shoulder so your right arm ends up behind you, with your left arm in front.

Roll your left shoulder back to reverse the movement. As you are rolling your left shoulder back, dip your left hip down and to the side as you transfer your weight from your right side to your left.

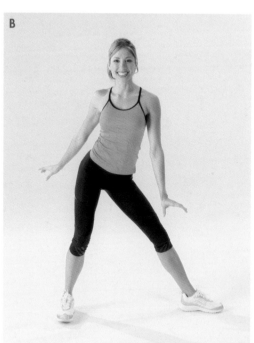

THE ROUTINE SO FAR

WARM-UP

16 steps in place = **MARCH**

8 steps out to the side = **MARCH OUT WIDE**

8 steps in place = **MARCH**

8 steps side to side = **STEP TOUCH SIDE TO SIDE**

4 steps forward = **TRAVEL UP**

4 steps back = **TRAVEL BACK**

8 steps side to side = **STEP TOUCH SIDE TO SIDE**

4 steps forward = **TRAVEL UP**

4 steps back = **TRAVEL BACK**

8 steps side to side = **STEP TOUCH SIDE TO SIDE**

8 steps side to side = **STEP TOUCH SIDE TO SIDE** (Low)

8 steps side to side = **STEP TOUCH SIDE TO SIDE**

4 steps forward = **TRAVEL UP**

4 steps back = **TRAVEL BACK** (Low)

4 steps forward = **TRAVEL UP**

4 steps back = **TRAVEL BACK** (Low)

4 steps forward = **TRAVEL UP**

4 steps back = **TRAVEL BACK** (Low)

8 steps side to side = **STEP TOUCH**

8 steps in place = **MARCH**

8 steps out to the side = **MARCH OUT WIDE**

STRETCH

2 arm circles = **ARMS UP STRETCH**

4 looks to the right,
4 looks to the left = **LOOK SIDE TO SIDE**

4 chins down, 4 chins up = **CHIN DOWN**

4 **CIRCLE NECK ROLLS**

1 arm circle = **ARMS UP**

3 flat back down,
2 round back up = **FLAT BACK DOWN**

6 single back staying down = **SINGLE BACK**

1 full body roll up = **RAG DOLL STRETCH**

1 arm circle = **ARMS UP STRETCH**

ISOLATION SEQUENCES

SHOULDER SIDE TO SIDE SIDE
4 to each side

GRAPEVINE
4 times to the right, 4 times to the left

PLIE 4 plies

PLIE WITH ARMS TO THE FRONT 4 plies

HAMSTRING STRETCH
2 stretches to each side

WIDE LEG STRETCH 2 stretches

PIVOT STRETCH
2 pivots to the right, 2 pivots to the left

SHAKE AND SHIMEE
4 shakes to the right, 4 shimees to the left

SIDE TO SIDE STRETCH
4 to the right, 4 to the left

SHOULDER ROLL
4 rolls to the right, 4 rolls to the left

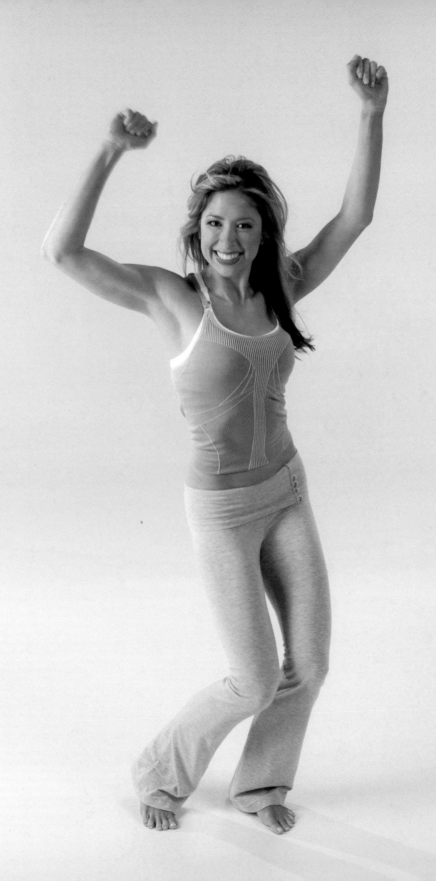

CHAPTER 4
THE MOVES

Congratulations! You've made it through the warm-up and now have arrived to the best part of the workout — the dance moves! Here are a few tips to keep you going:

- Don't be afraid to add a little bit of your own "flavor" to each move as you become more comfortable performing it (i.e. add another step in, shake your hips a little harder).

- Try each move 2 to 3 times for the first few workouts as you progress through the following chapter. Once you have the moves down pat, you can try the more advanced workout in Chapter 7.

- Switch up your music, you might want to try different styles to see which genre works best for you. To vary your routine, be daring and try on a different style each workout!

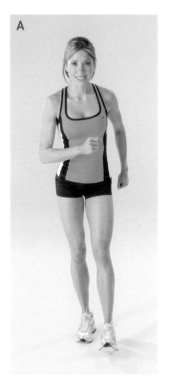

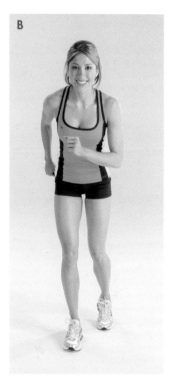

THE DANCE MOVES

MARCH FRONT AND BACK
(4 up, 4 back)

START POSITION: Stand with your feet close together, hands at your sides.

MOVEMENT:

A) Stepping forward, bring your left foot in front of you. Swing your right arm forward as you step.

B) Continuing to move forward, now bring your right foot in front of you. Swing your left arm forward as you step.

Continue to move forward for 4 steps, then reverse your direction and repeat, marching backwards until you reach your starting point.

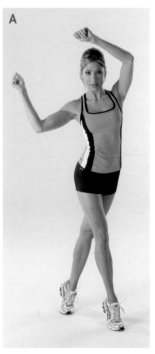

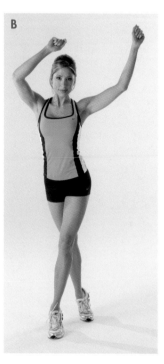

RUNWAY STRUT
(4 up, 4 back)

START POSITION: Stand with your feet close together, hands at your sides.

MOVEMENT:

A) Bringing your hands overhead, cross your right leg over your left as you begin to travel forward.

B) Immediately swing your left leg over your right as you continue traveling forward. Switch your hands to the opposite side as you do so. Keep alternating feet and hands as you move forward.

SIDE TAP
(side, together, side)

START POSITION: A) Stand with your feet close together, knees slightly bent, leaning forward from the hips. Arms are softly bent at the elbows.

MOVEMENT:

B) "Tap" your right foot out to your right side by extending your right leg from the hip, keeping most of your body weight on your left leg.

C) Bring your right leg back to your start position and repeat out to the same side. When you are done with your sequence, switch legs and repeat on the other side.

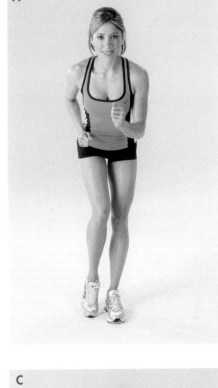

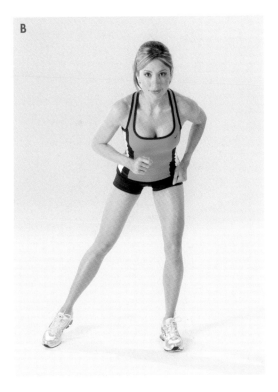

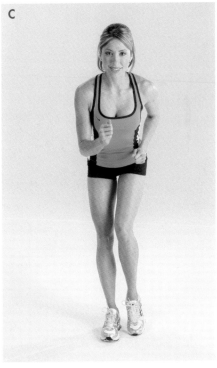

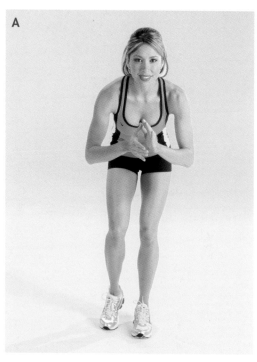

STEP TOUCH SIDE TO SIDE
ELONGATED *(side, together, side)*

START POSITION: A) Stand with your feet close together, knees slightly bent, leaning forward from the hips. Arms are softly bent at the elbows.

MOVEMENT:

B) Looking straight ahead, step out to your right side with your right leg. Keep your arms relaxed with your elbows softly bent at 90 degrees.

C) Stepping onto your right leg, complete the movement by lightly dragging your left leg across the floor to your right leg, then "touching" the floor next to your right foot with the ball of your left foot.

Repeat on the other side.

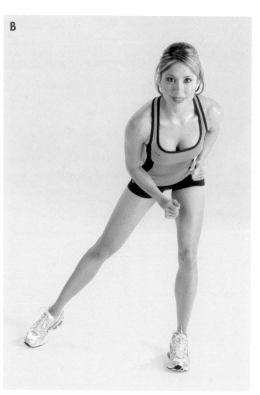

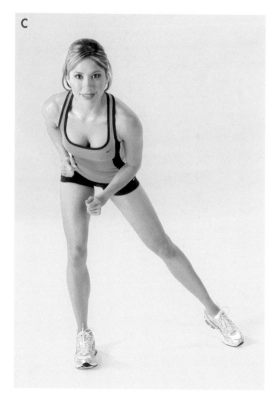

STEP SIDE WITH BACK TOUCH
(side, together, back)

START POSITION: (A, OPPOSITE) Stand with your feet close together, knees slightly bent, leaning forward from the hips. Arms are softly bent at the elbows.

MOVEMENT:

(B, OPPOSITE) Looking straight ahead, step out to your right side with your right leg. Keep your arms relaxed with your elbows softly bent at 90 degrees.

C) Stepping onto your right leg, complete the movement by bringing your left leg across, "touching" the floor behind you.

D) Reverse the movement and repeat on the other side.

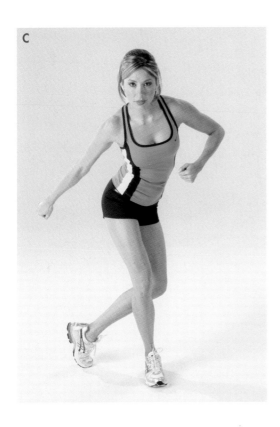

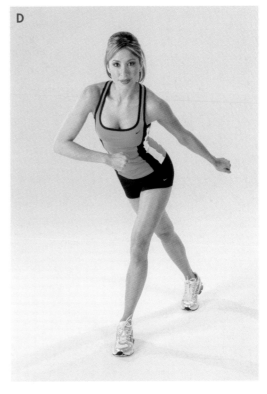

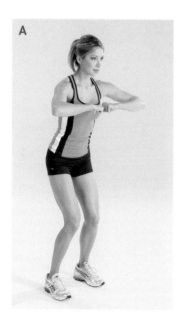

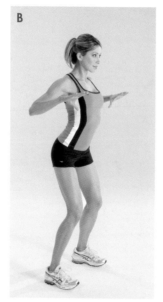

CHEST POPS
(front and back, front and back)

START POSITION: A) Stand with your feet shoulder-width apart and your knees slightly bent. Keeping your hands close to your chest, raise your elbows out to the side. Keep your chest up and your shoulders relaxed.

MOVEMENT:

B) In a slow, controlled fashion, lift your chest up and pull your shoulder blades together by bringing your elbows directly behind you. Once there, quickly return to your start position and repeat.

CHEST POPS WITH HIGH ELBOWS
(elbow right, elbow left, elbow right, elbow left)

START POSITION:

A) Stand with your feet close and knees slightly bent. Putting your hands in front of you, cross your right arm over your left wrist, keeping your left shoulder slightly down.

MOVEMENT:

B) In a slow, controlled fashion, lift your chest up and pull your shoulder blades together by bringing your elbows directly behind you. Once there, quickly return to your start position, crossing your left arm over your right hand, keeping your right shoulder slightly down.

C) Once again, lift your chest up and pull your shoulder blades together by bringing your elbows directly behind you. Reverse and keep repeating on each side.

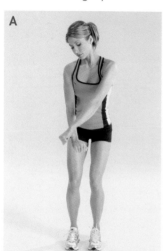

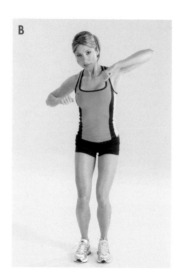

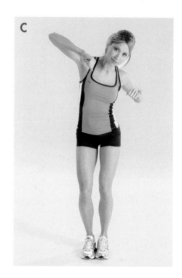

STOMP *(stomp right, stomp left, stomp right, stomp left)*

START POSITION: Stand with your feet close together, arms softly bent at the elbows.

MOVEMENT:

A) Looking straight ahead, step out to your right side with your right leg. As you are stepping, reach up with your right arm, grab the air above your head and "pull" down, while simultaneously "stomping" your left foot as you bring it in to meet your right leg.

B) Reverse the movement and repeat on the other side.

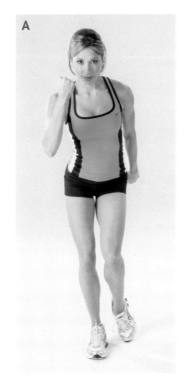
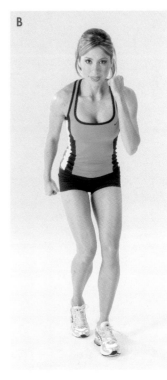

STEP SIDE TO SIDE

START POSITION: Stand with your feet close together, arms by your sides.

MOVEMENT:

A) Looking straight ahead, step out to your right side with your right leg. Keep your arms relaxed with your elbows softly bent at 90 degrees.

B) Stepping onto your right leg, complete the movement by bringing your left leg to your right leg, then quickly stepping back to the other side. Keep repeating on each side.

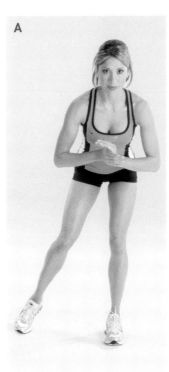
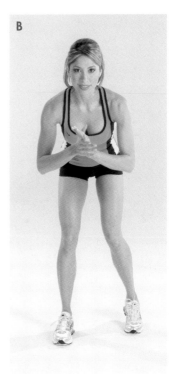

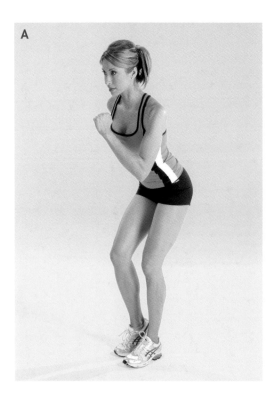

SINGLE ARM ROW
(row right, together, row left, together)

START POSITION: A) Stand with your feet close together, knees slightly bent, right arm back and left arm bent and forward.

MOVEMENT:

B) Stepping onto your right foot, extend your left leg back as you "row" your left arm forward.

C) As you bring your left leg back in, pivot on your right leg to face the other direction. Reverse the motion and repeat.

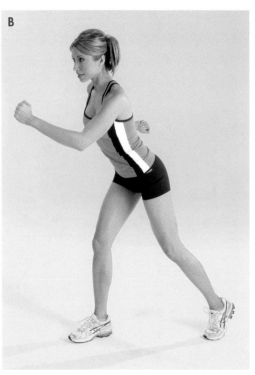

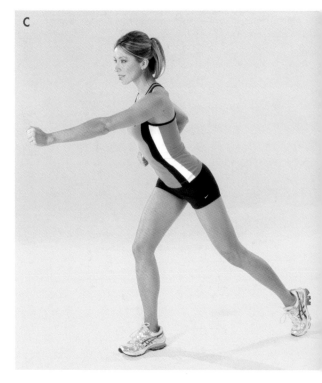

STEP STOMP

(step, stomp, bounce, step, stomp, bounce)

START POSITION: Stand with your feet close together facing a 45-degree angle. Hands are in the runner position.

MOVEMENT:

A) Step onto your right foot, picking your left foot up behind you. Lean slightly forward, leaving your hands in the runner's position.

B) Step back onto your left leg, lifting your right leg up.

C) As you bring your right leg down, pivot and face center. Add a small two-footed bounce, then switch your angle to the other side.

D) Now step onto your left foot, picking your right foot up behind you. Lean slightly forward, leaving your hands in the runner's position.

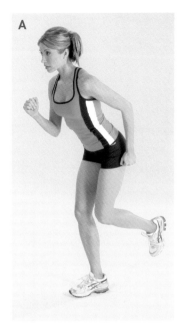
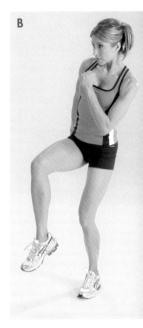

E) Step back onto your right leg, lifting your left leg up. Reverse direction and repeat the entire sequence.

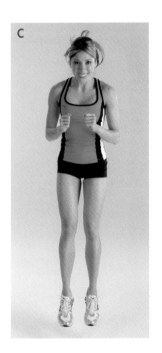
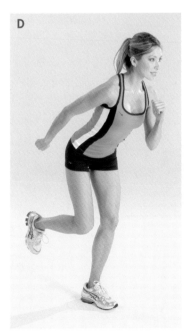
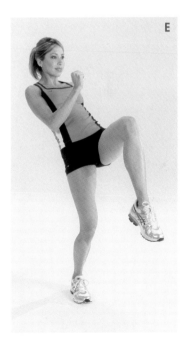

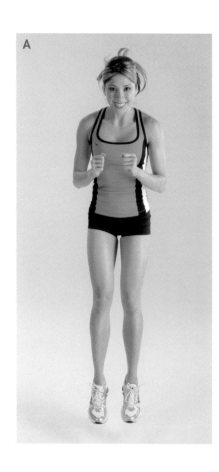

BOUNCE *(bounce, bounce)*

START POSITION: Stand with your feet close together, arms by your sides.

MOVEMENT:

A) Using your arms to help propel you, gently bend your knees and jump lightly. When landing, remember to bend your knees to cushion the impact.

SNAKE *(snake, snake, reverse, snake, snake, reverse)*

START POSITION: A) Stand with your feet close together, knees slightly bent, left arm back and right arm bent and forward.

MOVEMENT:

B) Stepping forward onto your left foot, "snake" your neck to the right as you straighten your left arm out. Bring your left arm in at the same time.

C) As you complete your "snake" movement with your neck, start pivoting back towards the left side

D) Once you pivot towards the left, step out with your left foot, letting your head and shoulders lead the way. Complete the motion by starting the sequence all over again on your left side.

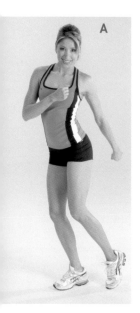

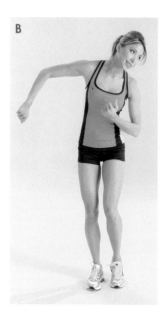

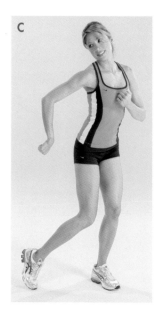

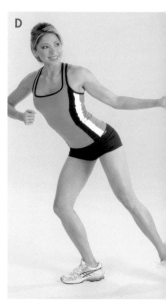

SWIM *(swim, swim, turn)*

START POSITION: Stand with your feet close together, hands by your sides, facing to the right.

MOVEMENT:

A) Bringing your arms up into the breast-stroke position, lift your right leg and step forward onto it.

B) As you step forward onto your right leg, complete the "swim" movement by pushing your hands straight out then around to your sides, as if you were "swimming" through water.

C) Bring both legs together and pivot to face the opposite direction.

D) Repeat traveling to the opposite side.

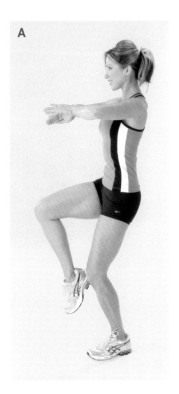

A

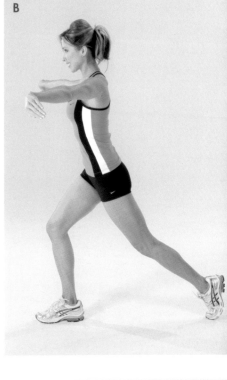

B

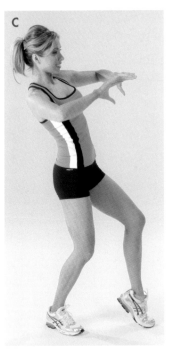

C

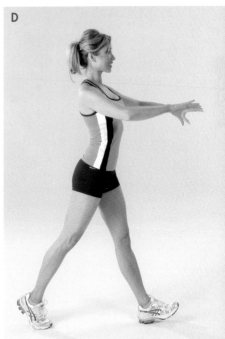

D

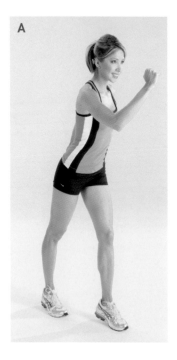

FRONT LEG KICK
(kick, step, tap)

START POSITION: A) Stand with your left leg front and right leg back, right arm front and left arm back.

MOVEMENT:

B) Kick your left leg forward, extending your arms straight.

C) Swing your right leg down in front of you, stepping directly onto it.

D) Shift your weight forward onto your right leg and "tap" the ground behind you with your left foot.

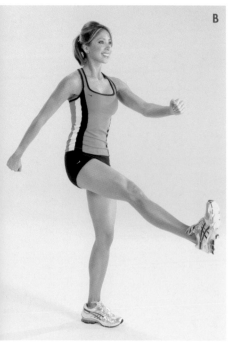

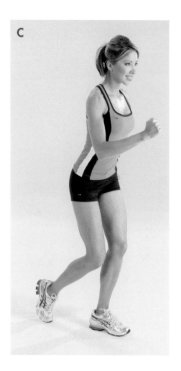

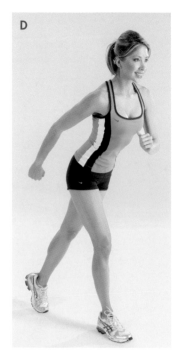

FRONT LEG KICK ADD ARMS

(kick, step, tap, arms)

START POSITION: A) Stand with your left leg front and right leg back, right arm front and left arm back.

MOVEMENT:

B) Kick your right leg forward, extending your arms straight and raising them up.

C) Step back onto your right leg.

D) Kick your left leg behind you. Extend your arms once again.

Bring your leg down, preparing to start the sequence over again with your right leg. Repeat.

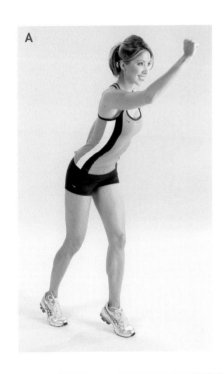

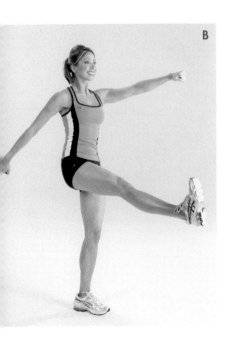

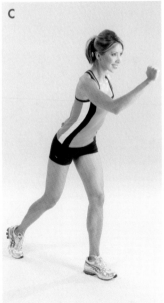

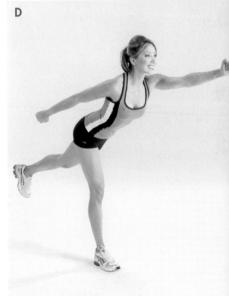

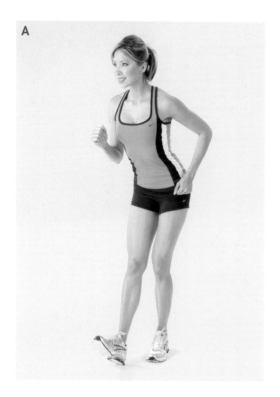

TRIPLE STEP
(step, step, back)

START POSITION: Stand with your legs close together, arms at your side.

MOVEMENT:

A) Step forward onto your right leg by bending at the hips and leaning slightly forward.

B) Bring your right leg back to center. Pick your left leg up and step it back, leaving your weight forward.

C) Quickly bring your left leg back to center, shifting your weight back onto your left leg and picking up your right foot. Repeat on the other side.

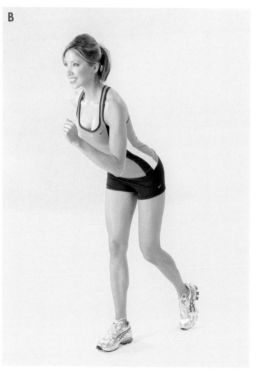

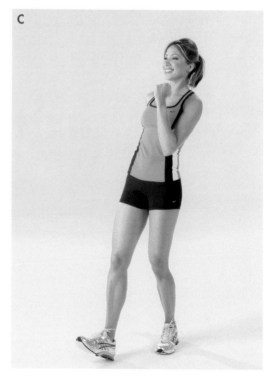

HIP HOP MOVE
(arms, arms, side)

START POSITION: Stand with your feet close together, arms softly bent at the elbows.

MOVEMENT:

A) Looking straight ahead, step out to your right side with your right leg. As you are stepping, bring your right arm out to the side as you bring your left arm in. Quickly reverse the movement 2 more times, effectively "triple-pumping" with your arms for every one step to the side you take.

B) Reverse the movement and repeat on the other side.

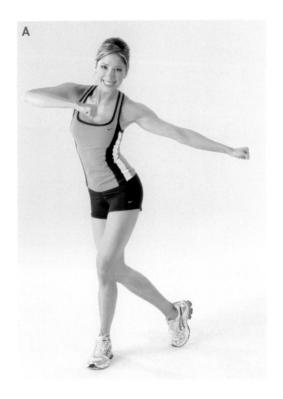

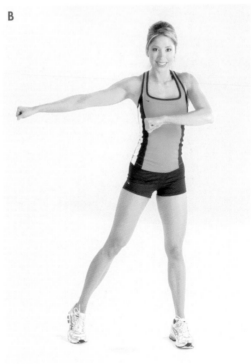

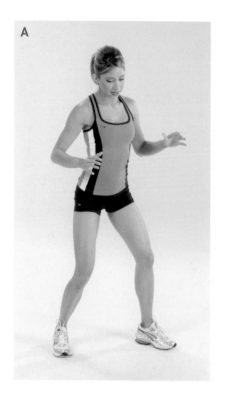

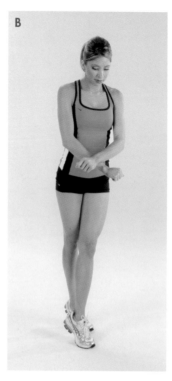

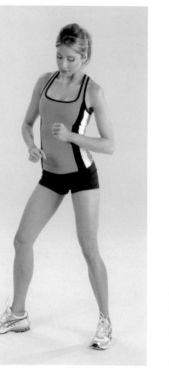

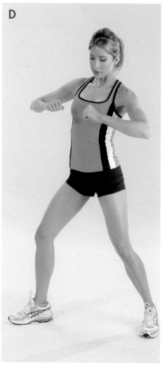

SCISSORS BOUNCE
(scissors, scissors, bounce, bounce)

START POSITION:
A) Stand with your feet wide apart, arms at the ready.

MOVEMENT:
B) Looking at the floor ahead of you, quickly jump to the right, crossing your feet as you land.

C) Uncross your feet and step out to the right by lightly jumping one more time. Hold that position for 2 counts, bouncing in place.

D) Variation with chest pops: In a slow, controlled fashion, lift your chest up and pull your shoulder blades together by bringing your elbows directly behind you. Once there, quickly return to your start position and repeat.

FUNKY FEET

(side-together-side, side-together-side)

START POSITION:

A) Stand with your feet close together, slightly leaning forward from your hips.

MOVEMENT:

B) Looking at the floor ahead of you, step out to the right, leaving your left leg in place.

C) Quickly slide your left leg half way over to your right leg.

D) Then immediately slide it back out to the left. Repeat on the other side.

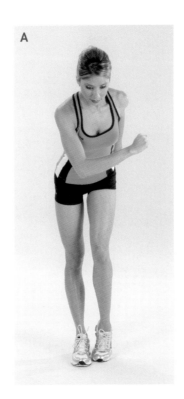

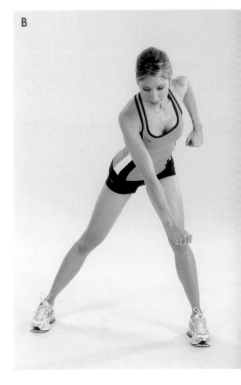

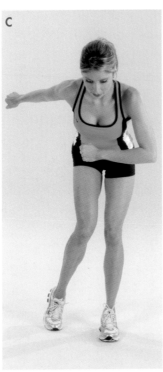

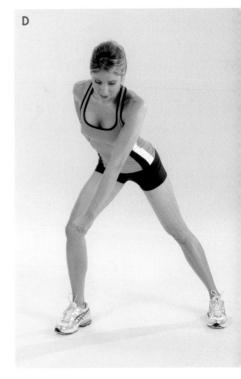

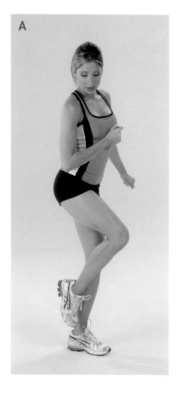

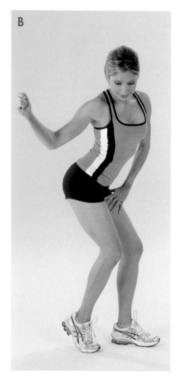

HIP ROCK SIDE TO SIDE *(hip and side, hip and side)*

START POSITION: Stand with your feet close together, arms relaxed at your sides, body at a 45-degree angle.

MOVEMENT:

A, B) Bringing your right leg and right arm up, step out by swinging your hip and arm to the right.

C) Keeping your knees bent and your torso slightly forward, begin to bring your weight over to your left side by pushing your hips to the back and left using a semi-circular motion as you pivot your body to the left side.

D) Once on your left, reverse the movement to repeat.

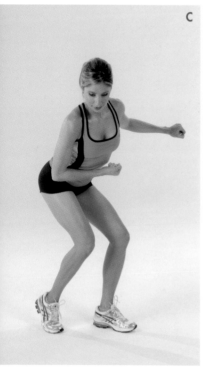

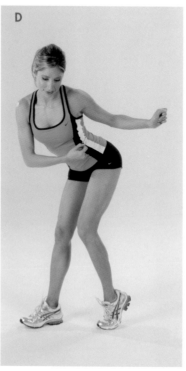

CIRCLE ARMS

(circle arms, circle arms)

START POSITION: Stand with your feet close together, hands at your sides.

MOVEMENT:

A) Bringing your hands overhead, step your right leg out directly in front of you.

B) Make two small circles in the air before fully extending your arms overhead.

C) Bring your left leg in, and pivot to repeat the movement in the opposite direction.

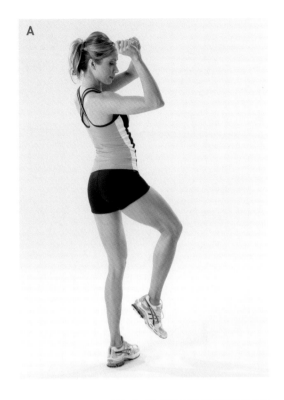

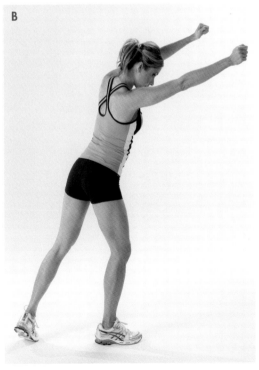

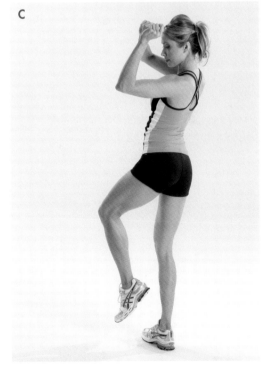

STEP IT BACK

(back-together-back, back-together-back)

START POSITION: Stand with your feet close together, hands at your sides.

MOVEMENT:

A) Step your right leg back at a 45-degree angle.

B) Bring your left leg back to meet your right leg.

C) Pivot and step back on your left, repeating the movement on the other side.

A
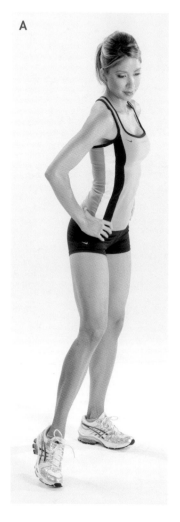

B
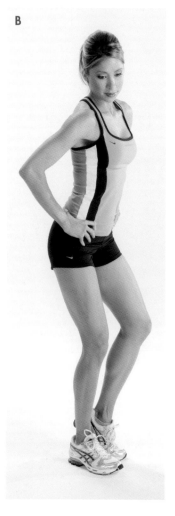

C
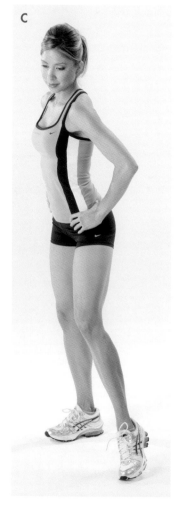

COWGIRL CIRCLE AROUND THE WORLD *(circle arms-turn, circle arms-turn)*

START POSITION: Stand with your feet close together, hands at your sides, body at a 45-degree angle.

MOVEMENT:

A) Bringing your hands overhead, step your left leg out directly in front of you.

B) Make one small half circle in the air with your arms before as you extend forward into the step.

C) Bring your left leg back as you complete the circle with your arms, pivoting one quarter-turn to repeat the movement to the next direction.

D) Continue repeating the movement until you have completed a full turn.

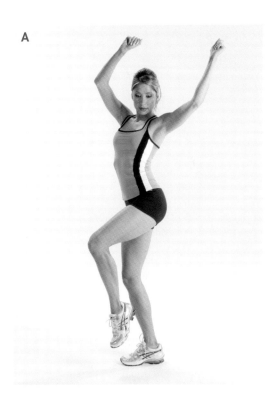

A

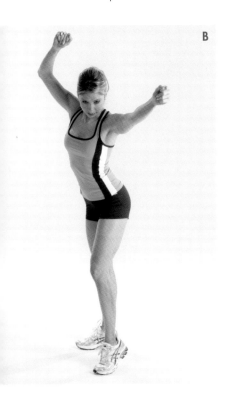

B

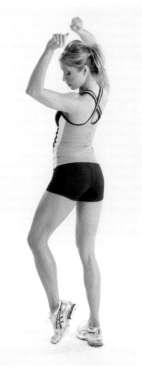

C

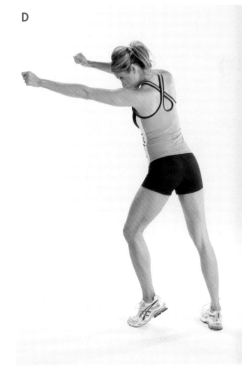

D

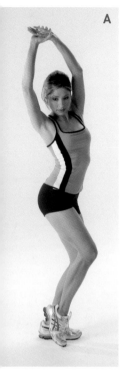 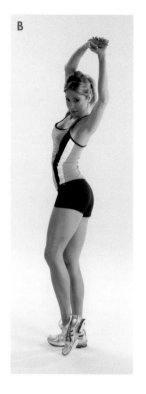 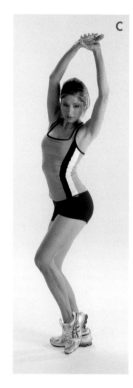

COWGIRL POP IT
(hip, hip, switch)

START POSITION: Stand with your feet close together, hands at your sides, body at a 45-degree angle.

MOVEMENT:

A) Bringing your hands overhead, pull your right leg up by rolling up onto the ball of your right foot.

B) Push your hip up by pivoting on the ball of your foot slightly.

C) Quickly return to your start position and repeat.

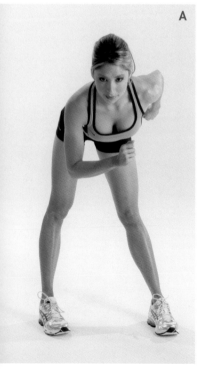 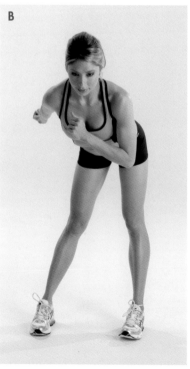

STRAIGHT LEGS, HIP BOUNCE
(bounce-bounce, side, bounce-bounce, side)

START POSITION: Stand with your feet wide apart, hands at your sides, leaning forward at a 45-degree angle.

MOVEMENT:

A) Lean all of your weight over to your right hip.

B) Quickly switch direction and lean to the left.

MAMBO

(cross heel-turn, cross heel-turn)

START POSITION: Stand with your feet together, hands at your sides.

MOVEMENT:

A) Cross your right heel in front of your left leg. Throw your right hip out to the side.

B) Pivot on your right heel as you switch direction by throwing your left hip out to the left side. Bring your right leg back, switch legs and repeat.

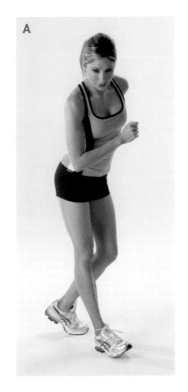
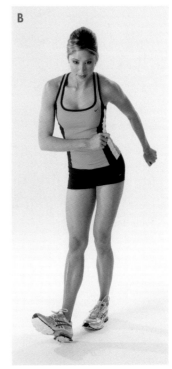

CHA CHA CHA

(cha, cha, cha)

START POSITION: Stand with your feet together, hands at your sides.

MOVEMENT:

A) Make an outward semi-circle with your right hip and knee by rolling on the ball of your right foot.

B) Placing your right foot down, switch to your left side and repeat.

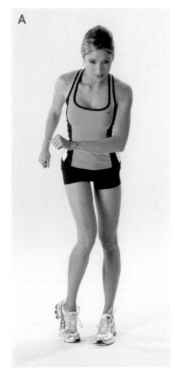
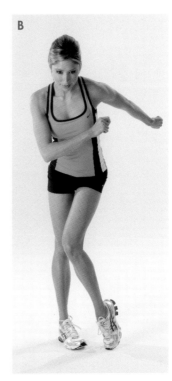

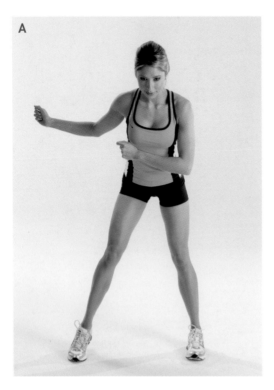

BOX STEP
(side, back, over, front)

START POSITION: Stand with your feet together, hands at your sides.

MOVEMENT:

A) Step out directly to your left.

B) Bring your right leg directly behind your left leg.

C) Cross your left leg over your right.

Bring your left leg forward to repeat the sequence.

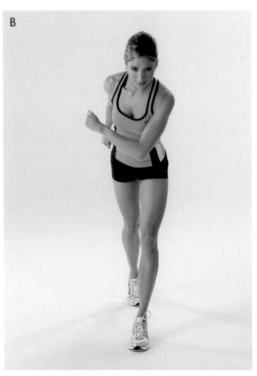

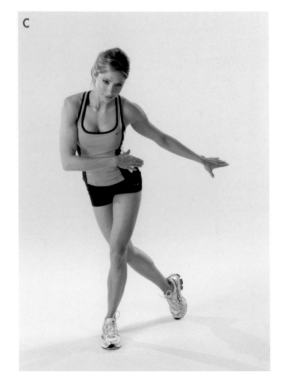

STEP BACK WITH HEAD TURN
(back and look, back and look)

START POSITION: A) Stand with your feet together, arms at the ready.

MOVEMENT:

B) Step directly back with your right leg, looking over your right shoulder as you extend your arms back.

C) Bring your right leg back to center. Switch sides and extend your left leg back while looking over your left shoulder.

Switch sides and repeat.

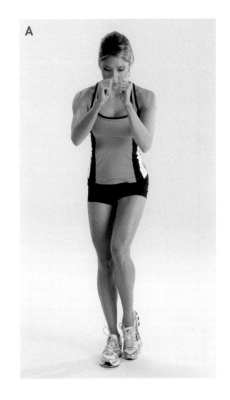

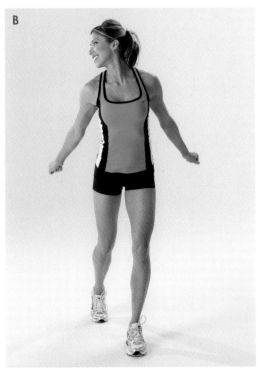

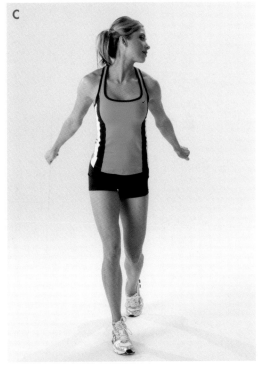

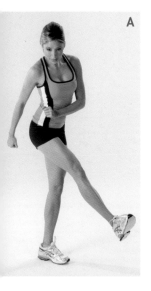
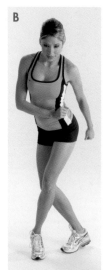
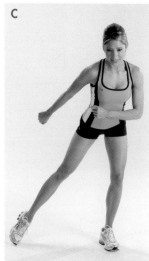

KICK CROSS TOUCH
(kick-cross-touch, kick-cross-touch)

START POSITION: Stand facing forward with your feet together, arms at the ready.

MOVEMENT:

A, B) "Kick" your right leg out and over to the left, crossing your left leg when you put it down.

C) Swing your left leg out from behind your right leg, "touching" the floor slightly behind you.

"Kick" your left leg out to reverse the motion and repeat on the other side.

SHAKE
(hips and shoulders, hips and shoulders)

START POSITION: Stand facing forward with your feet together, arms at the ready.

MOVEMENT:

A) Shift your weight to the left side, quickly pushing your right hip forward and lifting your right leg at the same time.

B) Stepping back onto your right leg, quickly reverse the movement and do the same as you shift your weight over to your left side.

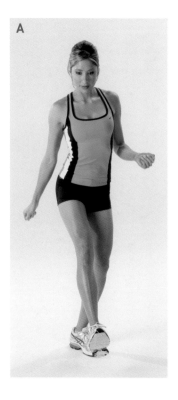
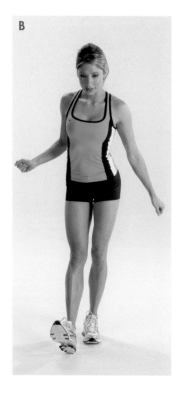

DIAGONAL PUMP

(pump-together-pump, pump-together-pump)

START POSITION: Stand with your feet close together, knees slightly bent. Arms are softly bent at the elbows.

MOVEMENT:

A) Step out to your right side with your right leg. Lift your left arm out to the side, slightly above your shoulder and bring your right arm in towards your chest as you do so.

B) Bringing your left leg over to meet your right leg, "pump" your arms by performing a chest pop (see page 62) at the same time.

C) Step out to the right to perform again.

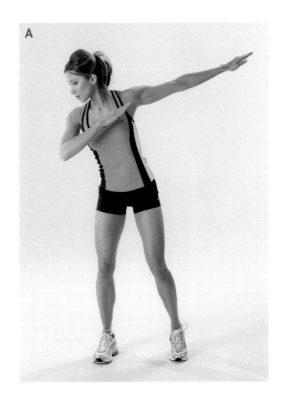

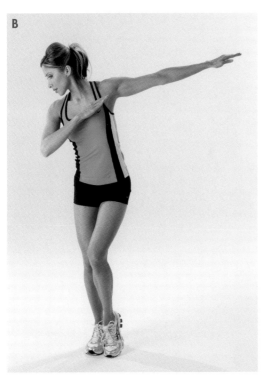

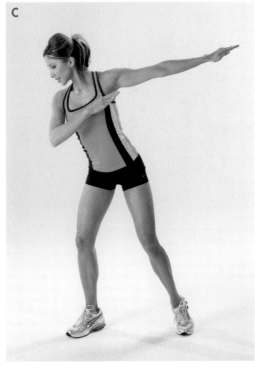

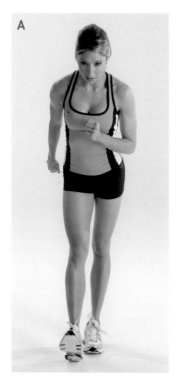
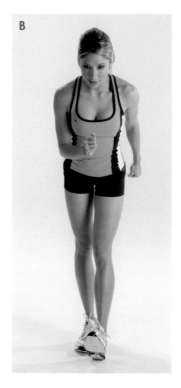

HEEL TAPS
(heel, heel)

START POSITION: Stand with your feet close together, knees slightly bent, arms at the ready.

MOVEMENT:

A) Tap your right heel in front of you. Lean forward slightly.

B) Bring back your right leg to your start position and extend your left leg out, tapping your left heel in front of you. Switch sides and repeat.

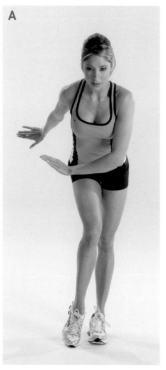
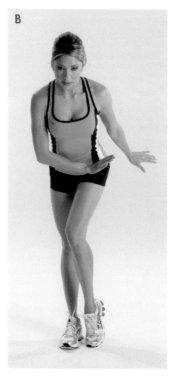

NEW SHOES
(toe and hip, switch, toe and hip)

START POSITION: Stand with your feet close together, knees slightly bent, arms at the ready.

MOVEMENT:

A) Tap the ball of your right foot in front of you. Lean forward slightly, with your weight distributed on your left side.

B) Bring your right leg back to your start position and lift your left leg to tap in front of you. Switch sides and repeat.

HOUSE IT

(chest pop, chest pop, hip pop, other side)

START POSITION: A) Stand with your feet shoulder-width apart and your knees slightly bent. Keeping your hands close to your chest, raise your elbows out to the side. Keep your chest up and your shoulders relaxed.

MOVEMENT:

B) Step out to your right. As you do so, perform a chest pop by lifting your chest up and pulling your shoulder blades together by bringing your elbows directly behind you. Quickly bring your feet together and repeat.

C) After the second chest pop, step to the right one more time, this time leaving your right leg out and rolling your knee inwards to "pop" your right hip. Bring your feet together and reverse direction.

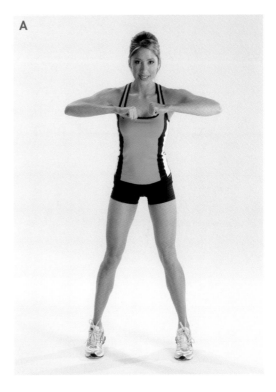

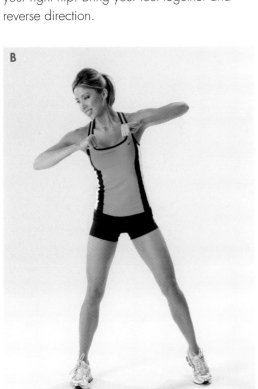

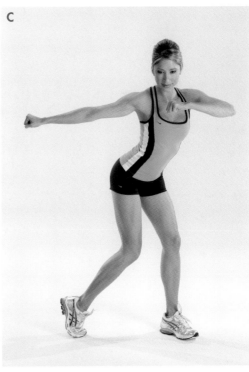

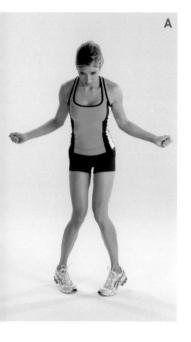
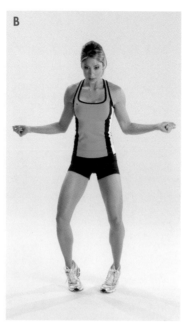

NOODLE LEGS
(up, up, back, back)

START POSITION: Stand with your feet shoulder width apart and your knees slightly bent. Keep your elbows bent and hands slightly out to the side. Keep your chest up and your shoulders relaxed.

MOVEMENT:

A) Hop forward onto the balls of your feet rolling your knees inward, creating a "noodle leg" effect.

B) Quickly hop forward again, this time rolling your knees to the outside

Reverse direction, hopping backwards.

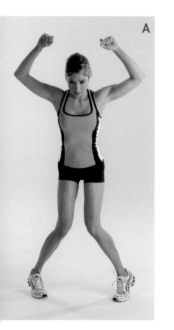
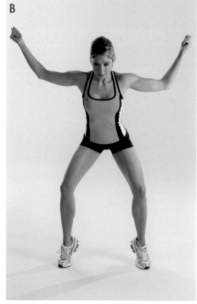

NOODLE LEGS
WIDE AND BACK
(up, up, back, back)

START POSITION: Stand with your feet hip-width apart and your knees slightly bent. Keep your elbows bent and hands slightly out to the side. Keep your chest up and your shoulders relaxed.

MOVEMENT:

A) Hop forward onto the balls of your feet rolling your knees inward, creating a "noodle leg" effect.

B) Quickly hop forward again, this time bringing your legs out wide. Roll your knees to the outside this time.

Reverse direction, performing the same movement, hopping backwards.

CHEST BOUNCES
(up, up, back, back)

START POSITION: A) Stand with your feet outside of your hip width, knees slightly bent. Keeping your hands close to your chest, raise your elbows out to the side. Keep your chest up and your shoulders relaxed.

MOVEMENT:

B) In a quick, controlled fashion, lift your chest up and pull your shoulder blades together by bringing your elbows directly behind you. At the same time, quickly bend your knees so that you "bounce" as pop your chest. Repeat.

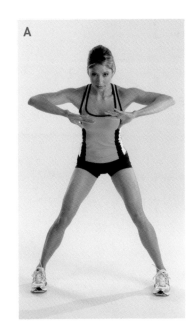
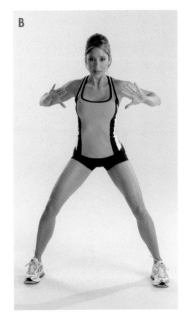

DANCE HALL QUEEN
(side, together, side)

START POSITION: Stand with your feet shoulder-width apart and your knees slightly bent. Keeping your hands close to your chest, raise your elbows out to the side. Keep your chest up and your shoulders relaxed.

MOVEMENT:

A) Step out to your right. As you do so, look to the right and bring both arms across your body to the left. Quickly bring your feet together and repeat.

B) After the second repetition, pivot on your feet to go to the left.

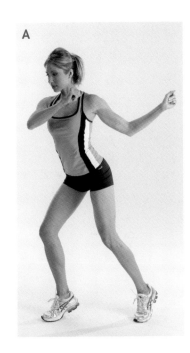
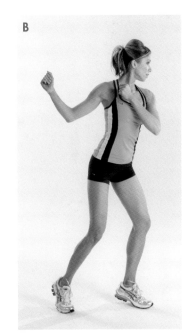

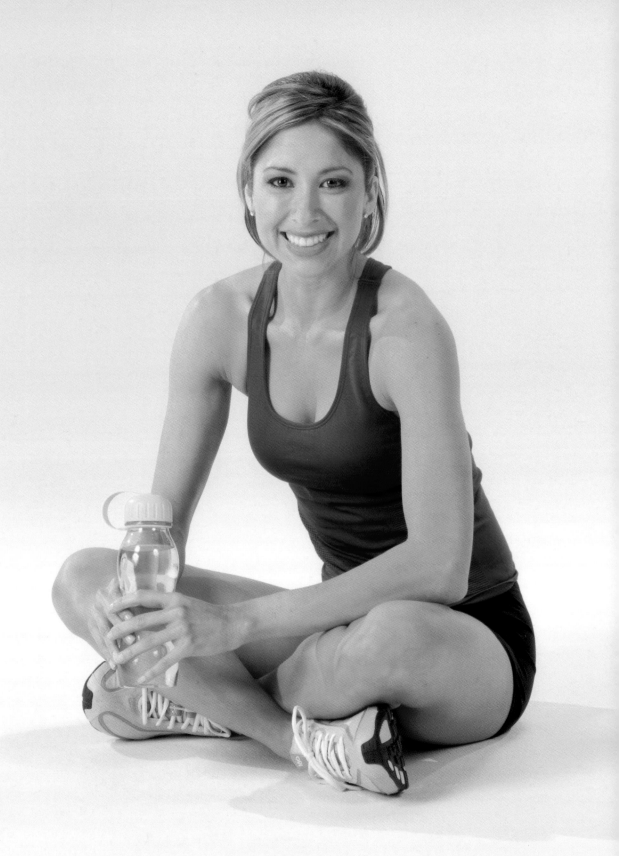

CHAPTER 5
THE COOL DOWN

The cool down part of your workout is the time to bring your heart rate back down, rehydrate and stretch out tired muscles. Your music selection should have a slower beat to help bring down your workout pace.

Remember to inhale gently at the start of the stretch movement, exhaling slowly as you feel the stretch deepen in your muscles.

COOL DOWN EXERCISES

ARMS OVERHEAD STRETCH *(2 times)*

START POSITION:
A) Stand with your feet shoulder-width apart, crossing your hands in front of your rib cage.

MOVEMENT:
B) Keeping your knees softly bent and your torso upright, make the motion of a circle by bringing your hands down towards the floor, out to your sides, finishing with palms facing out overhead.

Return your hands to their start position and repeat.

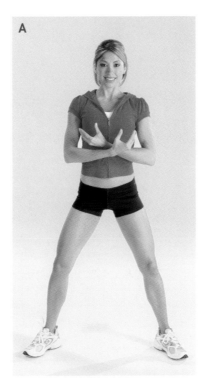
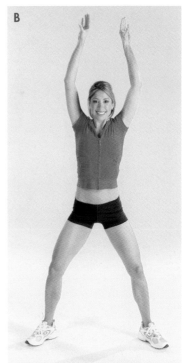

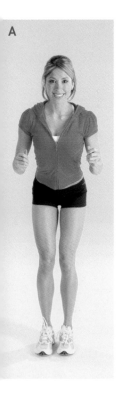

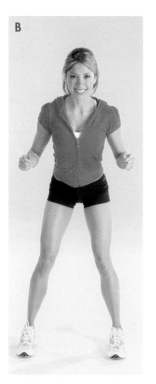

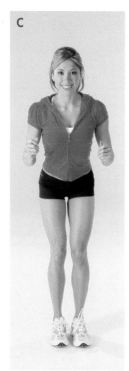

STEP TOUCH

(step, touch, step: 4 to the right, 4 to the left)

START POSITION: A) Stand with your feet close together, arms softly bent by your sides.

B) Keeping your head up and abdominals engaged, step out to your right, keeping your weight evenly distributed between both legs.

C) Bring your left leg over to your right leg, gently "touching" the floor next to your right leg with the ball of your left foot. Reverse the motion and repeat, this time traveling to the left side.

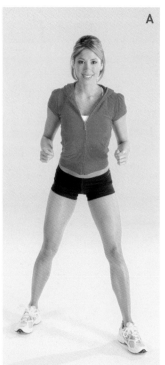

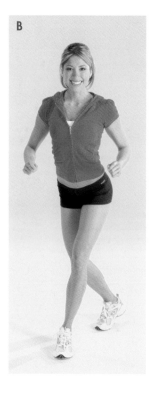

GRAPEVINE

(step, crossover, step, touch: 4 times to the right, 4 times to the left)

START POSITION: A) Stand with your feet shoulder-width apart, arms softly bent at the elbows.

MOVEMENT:
B) Cross your right foot over your left foot, traveling to the side.

Bring your back leg (left leg) out and to the side. Next, "touch" the floor next to your right leg with the ball of your left foot. Reverse direction and repeat on the other side.

MARCH
(16 steps in place)

START POSITION: Stand with your feet hip-width apart, arms by your sides.

MOVEMENT:

A) Keeping your head up and abdominals tight, raise your right leg by lifting your knee to hip height. Gently bring your left arm forward to eye level in a "swinging" motion, with your elbow softly bent at 90 degrees.

B) Return your left leg to the floor and repeat on the other side, being sure to alternate the arm motion as you raise the opposite leg. Reverse and repeat on the other side.

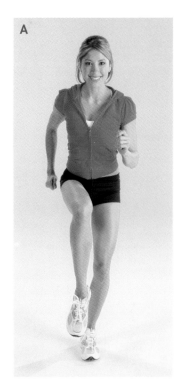
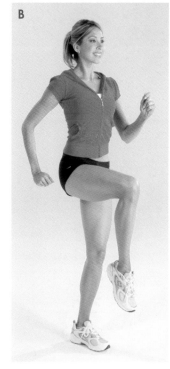

FLAT BACK DOWN
(3 down, 2 up)

START POSITION: A) Stand with your feet shoulder-width apart and your knees slightly bent. Lean forward 90 degrees at your hips, supporting your upper body by placing your hands on your thighs.

MOVEMENT:

B) In a slow, controlled fashion, round out your shoulder blades by dropping your chin to your chest and pulling your navel in as you lift your torso up towards the ceiling. Slowly roll up into a full upright position.

Reverse the movement by gently arching your back as you descend into the original start position. Repeat.

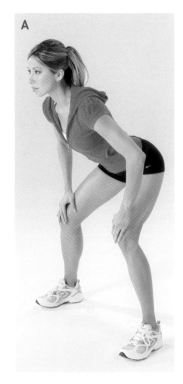
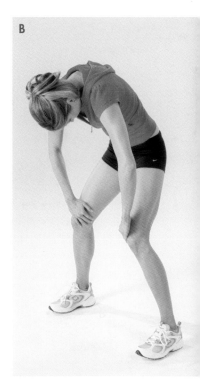

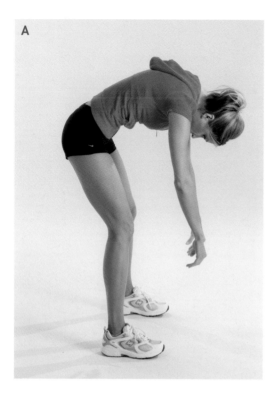

ROLL UP STRETCH
(1 full body stretch)

START POSITION: A) Standing with your feet hip-width apart and knees slightly bent, lean forward so that your hands are relaxed, hanging at knee height.

MOVEMENT:

B) Lifting from your shoulder blades, slowly roll your torso upright in a relaxed manner.

C) Once you are upright, finish the movement by rolling your shoulders back and lifting your chest so that your back arches slightly. Continue into your start position and repeat.

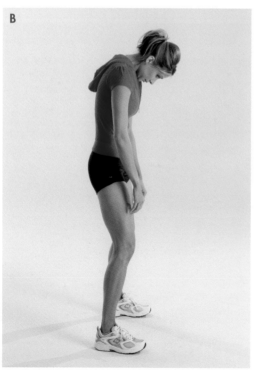

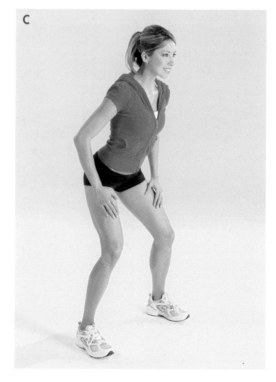

SHOULDER ROTATION
(1 full body stretch)

START POSITION: Stand with your feet wide apart, arms relaxed at your sides.

MOVEMENT:

A) While rolling your right shoulder forward and left shoulder back, lean towards your right side, slightly bending your knees.

B) Keeping your knees bent, bring your weight over to your left side by dipping your body down, then up, as you roll your right shoulder to your left side. Reverse the motion to repeat.

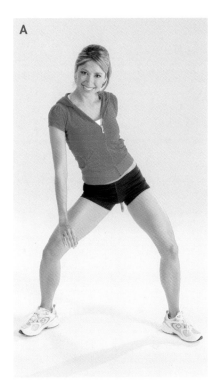
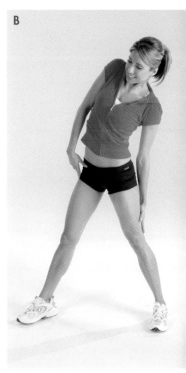

HIP ROCK
(1 full body stretch)

START POSITION: Stand with your feet wide apart, knees slightly bent, arms relaxed at your sides.

MOVEMENT:

A) Bringing your left shoulder forward and right shoulder back, lean over to your right side, distributing most of your weight on your right hip. Slightly bend your knees.

B) Keeping your knees bent, bring your weight over to your left side by dipping your body down, then up, as you raise your left shoulder to your right side. Reverse the motion to repeat.

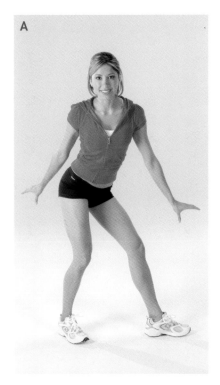
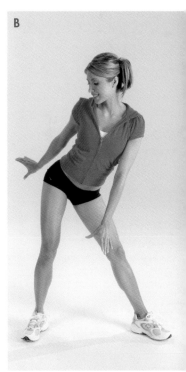

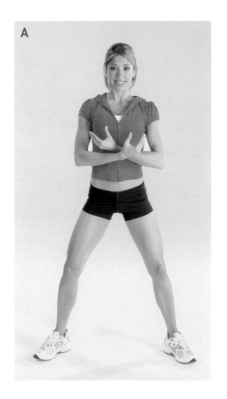

A

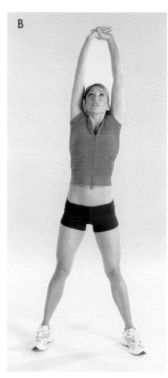

B

HALF-MOON STRETCH
(1 full body stretch)

START POSITION: A) Stand with your feet shoulder-width apart, crossing your hands in front of your rib cage.

MOVEMENT:

B) Keeping your knees softly bent and your torso upright, make the motion of a circle by bringing your hands down towards the floor, out to your sides, finishing with hands clasped overhead.

C) Leaving your hands clasped overhead and hips facing forward, gently lean slightly to your right.

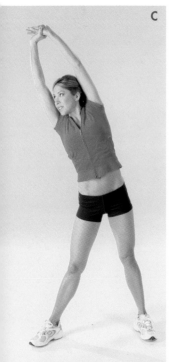

C

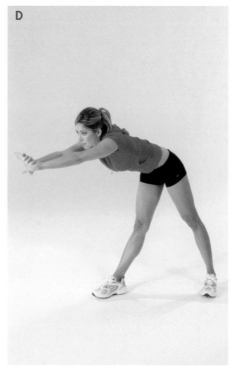

D

D) Pivot both legs to the right as your rotate your torso at the same time. Continue stretching forward until your torso is parallel to the floor, and both feet are pointing in the same direction.

E) Bring your torso and legs back to center by slowly pivoting your body. Once center, separate your hands and reach directly in front of you, elongating your stretch. Hold for a moment, then continue on to your left side.

F) Pivot both legs from center to the left as you rotate your torso at the same time. Clasp your hands together and

continue stretching forward.
Keeping your torso parallel
to the floor, make sure both
feet are pointing in the same
direction.

G) Leaving your hands
clasped, raise your torso
and arms upward until you
are almost upright. Reverse
direction and repeat.

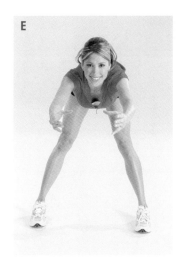

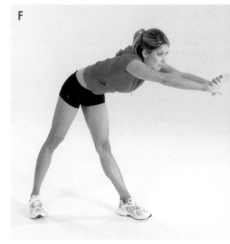

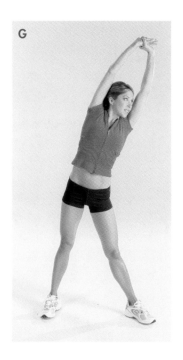

BALLET STRETCH
(1 full body stretch)

START POSITION: A) Pivot
both legs to the right as your
rotate your torso at the same
time. Stretch your arms and
torso forward, making sure your
upper body remains parallel
to the floor, and both feet
point in the same direction.

MOVEMENT:

B) Keeping your gaze ahead
and neck relaxed, softly
bring your right arm back,
leaving your left arm forward
in place. Hold for a few
seconds.

Bring your right arm back to
the front.

Bring your left arm back,
leaving your right arm
forward in place. Hold for
a few counts. Reverse the
movement and repeat.

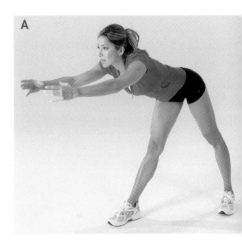

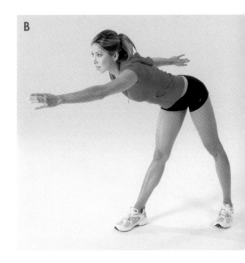

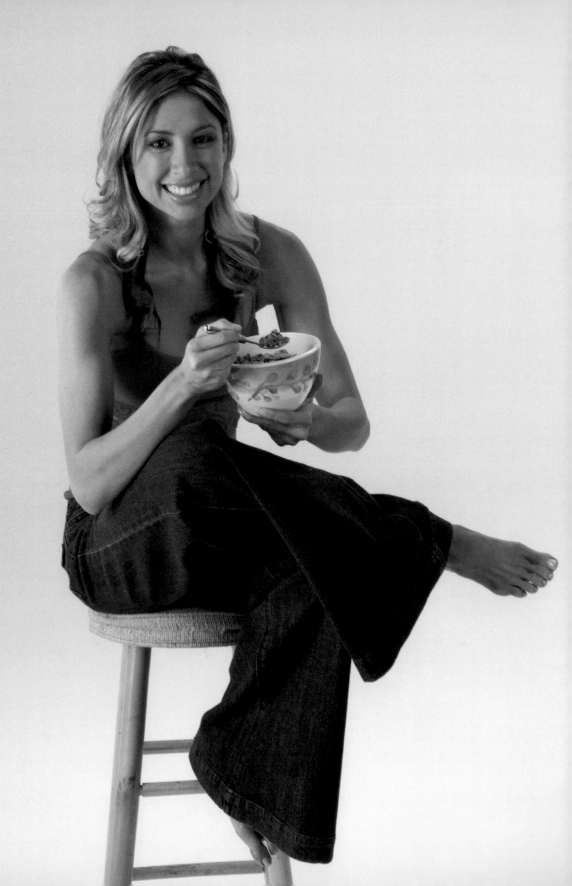

CHAPTER 6
14-DAY JUMP START MEAL PLAN

Is it all carbs and no fat or no carbs and all fat? High protein or low calorie? And what is all this about fiber? The world of diet and nutrition is confusing — and the rules seem to be constantly changing. So before we present you with ELLE Glam Fitness 14-day meal plan, we'll discuss some basic nutritional concepts, such as how to choose healthy carbs, why fiber is important and the benefits of drinking water. We'll also tell you why fad diets don't work and we'll provide you with the tools you need to create a healthy diet for optimal weight management.

This "diet" is a calorie controlled (1,300 to 1,400 calories) meal plan that provides an even balance of lean proteins, healthy carbohydrates and good fats. The meal plan offers three meals and two snacks daily and is loosely based on a Mediterranean-eating style (read: wine and olive oil, yes; trans fats and processed carbs, no). The Mediterranean diet has been shown to reduce the risk of many chronic diseases. This eating style is extremely flavorful and satisfying — it's definitely not about depriving yourself of delicious foods.

CARBOHYDRATES, FATS, PROTEIN: WHAT DOES IT ALL MEAN?

CARBOHYDRATES are the preferred fuel on which your body runs; in other words, they give you energy. The bad news is that if you take in too much of this energy, your body will "save it for later" in the form of fat. This is the theory that gave rise to low-carb diets. However, not all carbs are "bad." Fruits and vegetables are almost 100% carbohydrate ("almost" because fruits and veggies can also contain some protein and fat; for example, according to the USDA database, 100 grams of broccoli has 2.82 grams protein and .37 gram fat; 100 grams of banana has .33 gram fat and 1.09 grams protein), yet no diet would be healthy without these critical carbs. Other better known carbs include rice, potatoes, bread, cereal, pastas, sugar, candy and soda. A healthy diet includes mostly "good carbs," which are whole grains (such as brown rice and whole-wheat bread), fruits and vegetables. The term "bad carbs" (also called "simple carbs") refers to refined carbohydrates like candy, white bread, baked goods and refined starch such as white flour. These carbs earned their "bad" nickname due to the refining process that removes much of the healthy aspects of the food — such as fiber along with many vitamins and other nutrients.

A healthy, balanced diet will usually have 40 to 50% of its calories from carbohydrates. The majority of these calories should come from good carbs, while bad carbs and sugar should make up no more than 10% of your calories. Calories from bad carbs are believed to be a major cause of weight gain and are generally "empty calories," meaning they provide a lot of calories without any nutritional benefit.

PROTEINS are made up of amino acids that, when broken down, play a vital role in many bodily functions. In addition to keeping your body looking lean, proteins also play an important part in your immune system and your hormonal functions. A diet without enough protein would cause your body to break down its own muscle in order to obtain these vital amino acids, which would leave you with less lean body mass and less muscle tone.

Protein has gotten a bad rap because many foods that are high in protein are also high in saturated fat — think red meat, pork and full fat dairy. However, egg whites, skinless white meat poultry, soy based products, low-fat dairy, and fish are all lean, low-fat options. And while we tend to think of protein-rich foods as animal-based foods like poultry, red meat, and fish, even vegetarians can get plenty of proteins from such non-animal sources as nuts, beans, tofu, soy-based foods and protein powder.

Protein requirements are hotly debated among nutritionists and medical professionals; however, most agree that a diet that provides 25 to 35% of its calories from proteins is safe and healthy.

FAT in food, contrary to popular belief, does not directly contribute to fat on your body — so no, that muffin won't go directly to your thighs—and similarly, there is nothing magical about fat-free foods. The fact is, we all need fat in our diets. Fat fuels your body; it's the building block of hormones, and it's critically involved in your nervous system. In addition, healthy fats like olive oil and the fat in nuts are thought to make your skin look younger and more vibrant. And who doesn't want more of that?

"Bad fats" consist of trans fats and saturated fats. These fats have a bad rep because they're believed to directly contribute to heart disease, America's number one killer. Trans fats are found in many foods, including some margarines and some baked goods. New labeling laws make it mandatory for food companies to list the amount of trans fat contained in a food. You should aim to have 0 grams of trans fat in your food, as it is downright unhealthy.

Saturated fats are the fats found in foods like red meat, dairy, poultry skin and bacon. This fat is solid at room temperature, so you can actually see how much saturated fat is on your steak before it is cooked. Strive to get less than 10% of your calories from saturated fat.

"Good fats" are mono-unsaturated fats, which are believed to fight heart disease. These healthy fats are found in olives, olive oil, avocados, nuts, fish and flax seeds. As you'll see in the coming pages, we strive to incorporate many healthy fats in the ELLE Glam Fitness 14-day meal plan.

WHY FAD DIETS DON'T WORK

Fad diets tempt us with the promise of massive weight loss in a short amount of time; but while they may peel off the pounds in the short term, they rarely result in long-term weight loss. These diets usually omit entire food groups, leading to an imbalanced diet and little hope of lasting behavior change. After all, can you subsist on only grapefruit for the rest of your life, or without carbs of any kind? Fad diets may also result in binge eating and disordered eating patterns due to the nature of such extreme deprivation.

Instead of relying on a fad diet to drop pounds, try a calorie-controlled, balanced diet rich in lean proteins, complex carbs and healthy fats. If your nutrition plan is calorie controlled, and the nutrients are well balanced, you'll lose weight at a steady rate of 1 to 2 pounds per week — the optimal amount for healthy, long-term weight loss. The ELLE Glam Fitness 14-day plan provides you with roughly 1,300 to 1,400 calories per day, with very few calories coming from sugar and refined carbs. This healthy diet will make you feel energized — as opposed to fatigued and lethargic, which is how most fad diets will make you feel.

H2O: HYDRATE!

Water is the single most important nutrient required by your body, yet many of us quaff too little and walk around chronically dehydrated. Even mild dehydration can have profound effects of your body, leading to fatigue, water retention, poor muscle tone and decreased digestive efficiency.

HOW MUCH WATER DO YOU NEED?

You may have heard that 8 glasses of water per day is the gold standard; however, larger individuals and more active people may in fact require more water than that. A non-active person requires about ½ ounce of water for every pound of body weight. So, for a 150-pound person that would be 75 ounces of water per day — or about nine 8-ounce glasses per day. For an active, athletic person, the recommendation goes up to ¾ of an ounce of water for every pound of body weight. This means that the same 150-pound person needs about fourteen 8-ounce glasses per day! However, when figuring out your water requirements, keep in mind that everyone is different and that your body may need a little more or less than what these calculations suggest. Try starting with 64 ounces (or 8 glasses) per day, and then work your way up or down to your individual allowance.

TIPS FOR INCORPORATING ALL THAT WATER

Spreading your water intake throughout the day will help minimize trips to the bathroom. It's also best to start drinking water from the moment you wake in the morning. Aim to drink about 2 glasses each hour, with a minimum of 1 glass per hour. If you can stay within the range of 1 to 2 glasses per hour, you'll have no problem meeting your goal. You'll find that after a few weeks, your bladder will grow accustomed to this water intake and will require fewer trips to the bathroom.

GO WITH FIBER

Fiber is a material contained in plant-based foods that can't be fully digested by your body — and, believe it or not, this is a good thing! There are two categories of fiber: soluble and insoluble. Soluble fiber is best known for its ability to help reduce your cholesterol, and plays a starring role in such foods as oat bran, oatmeal, beans, peas, rice bran, barley, citrus fruits, strawberries and apple pulp.

Insoluble fiber gets its stellar reputation from its ability to keep your digestive tract running smoothly. Foods that are high in insoluble fiber include whole-wheat bread, wheat cereals, wheat bran, rye, rice, barley, most other grains, cabbage, beets, carrots, Brussels sprouts, turnips, cauliflower and apple skin.

Aim for a total of 25 grams of fiber per day. If your diet is rich in fruits, vegetables and whole grains, this allowance shouldn't be hard to achieve. As an example, here's the fiber content of some common foods:

1 fresh pear = 5 grams

1 cup blueberries = 3.5 grams

1 fresh orange = 3 grams

1 cup whole-wheat spaghetti = 6 grams

¾ cup bran flakes = 5 grams

1 slice whole-wheat bread = 6 grams

1 cup black beans = 15 grams

20 almonds = 3 grams

1 large carrot = 2 grams

1 cup corn = 4 grams

WAYS TO ADD FLAVOR WITHOUT CALORIES

Whether you're trying to lose weight or just "eat better," there are a few easy ways to add flavor to your food without tipping the calorie scales. Research has shown that foods with more flavor, and diets with more variety, are more likely to result in long-lasting weight loss. Below you'll find some everyday foods that can be used to kick up flavor without kicking up calories.

LEMON JUICE

Add a squirt of lemon to boost flavor in iced water, hot water or tea. You can also use it to dilute calorie-dense salad dressings. Lemon juice is practically calorie-free and offers a strong nutritional punch of vitamin C.

CHICKEN BROTH

Use chicken broth, or chicken bouillon, in place of butter or oil in many recipes to reduce the calories and fat. If a recipe calls for 4 tablespoons of butter, for example, try using only 2 tablespoons of butter and about ¼ cup of chicken broth. You'll save many calories and find that the flavor is just as good, if not better.

HERBS

Herbs such as basil, rosemary and thyme can be used in almost any dish to enhance the flavor, without adding calories. Chop them into soups, stews, marinades, steamed veggies and salad dressings, or sprinkle them on top of salads.

SPICES

Like herbs, spices can add a new flavor dimension sans calories. Try sprinkling cinnamon or nutmeg on your oatmeal, coffee, yogurt or cottage cheese.

LOW-SODIUM SOY SAUCE

Reduced-sodium soy sauce is packed with flavor but has almost no calories. You can sprinkle it on steamed vegetables, into a stir-fry or even on a salad. Even in the low-sodium version, the level of sodium is pretty high, though, so this may not be a great condiment for you if you're on a sodium-restricted diet.

EAT, DON'T SKIP

The ELLE Glam Fitness 14-day meal plan offers 3 meals and 2 snacks per day. It's critical to eat all of these meals and most of the snacks to ensure steady, healthy weight loss that will have you feeling healthy and energized all the while. Eating small, frequent meals will prevent you from getting too hungry, which could lead to an ice-cream binge. That will also give you optimal energy for daily activities and exercise. If you skip meals — especially breakfast — your body will go into "starvation mode," slowing your metabolism and making it even more difficult to lose those stubborn fat deposits.

14-DAYS MEAL PLAN

DAY 1

BREAKFAST: BERRY-NUT OATMEAL
Cook ½ cup dry oatmeal oats with ½ cup skim milk and ½ cup water; when cooked, add ½ tsp cinnamon, ¾ cup mixed berries and 2 tbsp chopped walnuts.

LUNCH: GRILLED CHICKEN AND GRAPE SALAD
In a large bowl, combine 2 cups mixed lettuce, 5 halved cherry tomatoes, ½ cup sliced mushrooms, ½ cup sliced cucumber, ¼ cup alfalfa sprouts, 8 halved grapes and 4 ounces sliced white meat chicken. Drizzle the salad with 1 tsp olive oil and a splash of vinegar. Serve with ½ of a 6-inch whole-wheat pita bread.

SNACK: BANANA YOGURT
6 ounces low-fat plain yogurt (Greek or regular) with ½ sliced banana mixed in.

DINNER: GRILLED TILAPIA WITH STRING BEANS AND WHOLE-WHEAT COUSCOUS
Combine 1 sliced medium tomato with 1 sliced red onion and sprinkle with 2 tbsp low-fat feta cheese and 2 tbsp light vinaigrette dressing. Grill a 5-ounce Tilapia filet (or other white flaky fish) with fresh herbs (such as parsley or rosemary). Serve the fish with 1 cup string beans (sautéed in 2 tsp olive oil) and ½ cup cooked whole-wheat couscous tossed with lemon juice and sliced scallions.

DAILY NUTRITION INFORMATION

1,378 calories

104 grams protein

153 grams carbohydrate

44 grams fat

27 grams fiber

EVENING SNACK: FRESH FRUIT
1 sliced peach.

DAY **2**

BREAKFAST: GOAT CHEESE OMELET

In a non-stick skillet with cooking spray (or with a splash of olive oil) make an omelet with 3 egg whites, 1 yolk and 1 ounce goat cheese. Serve the omelet with 1 slice wheat toast and 1 cup melon balls.

LUNCH: TUNA PITA

Mix 5 ounces water-packed tuna with 1 tbsp light mayonnaise and stuff into ½ of a 6-inch whole-wheat pita. Serve with an arugula salad composed of 1 cup washed and trimmed arugula, 1 tbsp chopped walnuts and 5 halved cherry tomatoes, dressed with 1 tsp olive oil and red wine vinegar, sea salt and freshly ground pepper.

SNACK: APPLE AND HUMMUS

1 small sliced apple dipped into 2 tbsp prepared hummus.

DINNER: WHOLE-WHEAT PASTA WITH MIXED VEGETABLES

Mix ¾ cup of cooked whole-wheat pasta with ½ cup of tomato sauce and 1 cup mixed steamed vegetables (such as broccoli, string beans, carrots, peas). Top with ¼ cup grated part-skim mozzarella cheese. Serve with a large green salad composed of romaine lettuce, 1 chopped tomato, ½ sliced cucumber and bell pepper, dressed with 2 tbsp low calorie vinaigrette.

EVENING SNACK: BERRIES AND CREAM

½ cup fresh mixed berries topped with 1 tsp non-dairy whipped topping.

DAILY NUTRITION INFORMATION

1,278 calories

91 grams protein

151 grams carbohydrate

40 grams fat

32 grams fiber

DAY **3**

BREAKFAST: PEACH PARFAIT

In a cereal bowl, layer 8 ounces of low-fat plain yogurt (Greek or regular), 1 sliced peach and 3 tbsp low-fat granola.

LUNCH: MEDITERRANEAN SALAD

In a large bowl, combine 2 cups mixed greens with 1 chopped tomato, ½ cup sliced cucumber, ½ cup sliced white mushrooms, ¼ cup chopped red pepper, ¼ cup chopped red onion, ⅓ cup canned black beans, ⅓ cup canned chickpeas and 3 black olives. Dress the salad with 2 tbsp light vinaigrette salad dressing and serve with 1 small whole-grain dinner roll.

SNACK: COTTAGE CHEESE AND FRUIT

Mix 1 cup 2% cottage cheese with ½ cup fresh fruit salad.

DINNER: TURKEY BURGER AND BROCCOLI

Grill or bake a 5-ounce turkey burger (use 99% fat-free ground turkey breast) and top with 1 cup sautéed mushrooms and onions made in 1 tsp olive oil. Serve with 1 cup steamed broccoli and 1 small baked sweet potato topped with 1 tbsp low-fat sour cream. Serve with 1 slice of tomato and 2 or 3 slices of cucumber, dressed with low-calorie vinaigrette dressing.

EVENING SNACK: WATERMELON CUBES

1 cup watermelon cubes.

DAILY NUTRITION INFORMATION

1,317 calories

96 grams protein

176 grams carbohydrate

34 grams fat

31 grams fiber

DAY 4

BREAKFAST: CEREAL AND BERRIES

In a cereal bowl, combine ¾ cup high-fiber cereal (such as bran flakes or All-Bran or Fiber One), 1 tbsp slivered almonds, ½ cup sliced strawberries and 1 cup skim milk.

LUNCH: ROASTED CHICKEN AND GOAT-CHEESE WRAP

In a whole-wheat wrap, spread 1 tsp honey mustard, then layer 4 ounces sliced white meat chicken with shredded romaine lettuce, ⅛ sliced avocado, 2 slices red onion and ¼ cup alfalfa, and sprinkle with 1 ounce of goat cheese. Wrap it up and serve.

SNACK: APPLE AND HUMMUS

1 small sliced apple dipped into 2 tbsp prepared hummus.

DINNER: GRILLED SHRIMP WITH SPINACH AND BROWN RICE

Grill (or bake) 5 to 6 ounces of shrimp with fresh herbs (such as parsley or thyme) and serve atop ½ cup cooked brown rice. Serve with 1 cup sautéed spinach (sauté in 1 tsp olive oil and minced garlic) and a sliced tomato and cucumber salad topped with 2 tbsp low-fat feta cheese and drizzled with 2 tbsp light vinaigrette dressing.

EVENING SNACK: FRESH FRUIT

1 sliced nectarine.

DAILY NUTRITION INFORMATION

1,334 calories

99 grams protein

164 grams carbohydrate

42 grams fat

38 grams fiber

DAY 5

BREAKFAST: PITA AND COTTAGE CHEESE
Spoon ½ cup 2% cottage cheese into a 6-inch warm whole-wheat pita; add a few slices of tomato. Serve with ¾ cup mixed berries.

LUNCH: DIJON TUNA SALAD
Combine 5 ounces water-packed white meat tuna with 1 stack of celery (chopped), ⅓ chopped green peppers, 1 tbsp Dijon mustard and 1 tbsp low-fat mayonnaise. Scoop Dijon tuna onto large mixed green salad composed of mixed greens, 1 cup red and green pepper strips, ½ sliced cucumber and 5 cherry tomatoes.

SNACK: BANANA-HONEY YOGURT
Mix 6 ounces low-fat plain yogurt (Greek or regular) with ½ sliced banana, then drizzle with 1 tsp honey.

DINNER: ROTISSERIE CHICKEN AND COUSCOUS
Combine 5 ounces of skinless white meat rotisserie chicken with 1 cup cooked whole-wheat couscous. Toss the chicken and couscous with 1 tsp raisins and 1 cup sautéed spinach (sauté the spinach in 2 tsp olive oil and minced garlic).

EVENING SNACK: STRAWBERRIES AND RICOTTA CHEESE
½ cup sliced strawberries with 1 tbsp non-fat ricotta cheese and sweetener (if desired).

DAILY NUTRITION INFORMATION

1,337 calories

127 grams protein

144 grams carbohydrate

31 grams fat

25 grams fiber

DAY **6**

BREAKFAST: BANANA-NUT OATMEAL
Cook ½ cup raw oats with 1 cup skim milk. Add ½ tsp cinnamon, ½ sliced banana and 3 tbsp chopped walnuts to cooked oats.

LUNCH: VEGGIE WRAP
Fill a whole-wheat wrap with 2 tbsp prepared hummus, 1 cup mixed greens, 1 medium chopped tomato, ½ cup sliced cucumber, ½ cup sliced white mushrooms and ¼ cup chopped red pepper. Serve with 5 baby carrots and 1 piece part-skim mozzarella string cheese.

SNACK: PEANUT BUTTER CELERY STALKS
Fill 3 celery stalks with 2 tbsp all-natural peanut butter.

DINNER: BEEF KEBAB AND BROWN RICE
Thread 4 ounces of grilled (or baked) sirloin cubes on shish kebab skewers with roasted red and green peppers cubes, zucchini and mushrooms, alternating between the different vegetables. Serve with ½ cup cooked brown rice and a salad made of 1 cup salad greens with ¼ cup chopped tomato, ¼ cup diced cucumber and ¼ cup diced red bell pepper. Dress with 2 tbsp light vinaigrette dressing.

EVENING SNACK: MELON BALLS
1 cup melon balls with a twist of lemon.

DAILY NUTRITION INFORMATION
1,370 calories
94 grams protein
153 grams carbohydrate
52 grams fat
27 grams fiber

DAY **7**

BREAKFAST: POACHED EGGS AND ASPARAGUS
Poach 2 eggs and steam 4 asparagus spears. Place eggs and asparagus in ½ whole-wheat English muffin. Serve with ½ medium grapefruit.

LUNCH: CHOPPED FETA AND APRICOT SALAD
In a large bowl, combine 2 cups salad greens with 1 ounce low-fat feta cheese, 5 dried apricot halves, ½ cup sliced cucumber, ½ cup chickpeas and 2 tsp chopped walnuts. Dress with 2 tbsp light vinaigrette dressing. Serve with ¼ of a 6-inch whole-wheat pita.

SNACK: CRACKERS AND PEANUT BUTTER
Spread 1 tbsp all-natural peanut butter on 3 whole-wheat crackers.

DINNER: BBQ TURKEY AND BROCCOLI
Grill (or bake) 5 ounces of skinless white meat turkey breast brushed with 1 tbsp BBQ sauce. Serve with 1 cup sautéed broccoli florets (sautéed in 1 to 2 tsp olive oil and minced garlic) and a tossed green salad dressed with 2 tbsp light vinaigrette dressing.

EVENING SNACK: FROZEN YOGURT
½ cup non-fat frozen yogurt.

DAILY NUTRITION INFORMATION

1,311 calories

91 grams protein

120 grams carbohydrate

56 grams fat

26 grams fiber

DAY **8**

BREAKFAST: CEREAL AND STRAWBERRIES
In a cereal bowl, combine ¾ cup high-fiber cereal (such as bran flakes or All-Bran or Fiber One), 1 tbsp slivered almonds, ½ cup strawberries and 1 cup skim milk.

LUNCH: TURKEY, AVOCADO AND ARUGULA PITA
Stuff ½ of a 6-inch whole-wheat pita with 4 ounces turkey breast, ¼ cup sliced avocado, ½ cup trimmed arugula and 1 tsp Dijon mustard. Serve with 1 medium sliced apple.

SNACK: VEGETABLES AND CHEESE
8 baby carrots, 5 cherry tomatoes and 1 piece part-skim mozzarella string cheese.

DINNER: HERB GRILLED SWORDFISH
Brush a 5-ounce swordfish steak with 1 tbsp olive oil and season with sea salt, fresh ground pepper and ¼ cup chopped fresh herbs (such as basil, rosemary or thyme). Marinate in refrigerator, for a minimum of ½ hour and a maximum of 4 hours. Grill (or bake) swordfish until cooked through. Serve with 10 steamed asparagus spears and 1 small baked potato.

EVENING SNACK: BERRIES AND CREAM
½ cup fresh mixed berries with 1 tsp non-dairy whipped topping.

DAILY NUTRITION INFORMATION

1,330 calories

96 grams protein

151 grams carbohydrate

48 grams fat

41 grams fiber

DAY **9**

BREAKFAST: WAFFLE AND BLUEBERRIES

Top 1 whole-grain toasted waffle with 1 cup blueberries, 4 tbsp low-fat yogurt and 1 tsp honey.

LUNCH: MEDITERRANEAN SHRIMP SALAD

In a salad bowl, combine 4 ounces of grilled (or boiled) shrimp with 3 tbsp crumbled feta cheese. Pile shrimp and cheese mixture on a bed of mixed salad (2 cups romaine lettuce, ½ sliced peppers, ¼ sliced cucumbers and ½ cup sliced mushrooms). Dress the salad with 2 tbsp light vinaigrette dressing and serve with 4 whole-wheat crackers and 1 small nectarine.

SNACK: WHEAT PRETZELS

2 ounces whole-wheat pretzels.

DINNER: CHICKEN, BABY SPINACH AND TOMATO SALAD

Marinate in refrigerator, for a minimum of ½ hour and a maximum of 12 hours, a 5-ounce boneless skinless chicken breast in 1 tsp lemon juice and 1 tsp olive oil. Season with a dash of sea salt, fresh ground pepper and dried parsley to taste. Sauté chicken in non-stick skillet or grill pan (sprayed with cooking spray) until cooked through. Pile 2 cups baby spinach on a plate and top with chicken, 1 sliced tomato, ½ sliced cucumber, 2 tsp shredded Parmesan and a drizzle of balsamic vinegar.

EVENING SNACK: PURÉED FRUIT

½ cup unsweetened apple sauce or puréed apricots or pears.

DAILY NUTRITION INFORMATION

1,263 calories

94 grams protein

450 grams carbohydrate

37 grams fat

24 grams fiber

DAY **10**

BREAKFAST: YOGURT-HONEY CRUNCH
In a small bowl, combine 8 ounces non-fat plain Greek yogurt with
1 tsp honey, ½ cup blueberries and ½ cup high-fiber cereal.

LUNCH: TOMATO MOZZARELLA SALAD
Layer 1 sliced medium tomato with 3 ounces sliced fresh mozzarella
cheese and ½ cup shredded arugula or mixed greens. Drizzle salad
with 1 tsp olive oil, balsamic vinegar, sea salt and ground pepper to
taste. Serve with ½ of a 6-inch warm whole-wheat pita bread.

SNACK: TURKEY ROLL UP
Roll up 3 ounces deli turkey slices with 1 ounce low-fat cheddar.

DINNER: VEGGIE PIZZA
Top 2 slices of purchased thin crust pizza (or 1 slice of regular crust
pizza) with 1½ cups mixed vegetables (such as mushrooms, peppers,
onions, spinach, eggplant). Serve with green salad (1 cup mixed greens,
¼ cup chopped tomato, ¼ cup diced red pepper, ¼ cup shaved
carrots) topped with 2 tbsp slivered almonds and dressed with 2 tbsp
light vinaigrette dressing.

EVENING SNACK: FRUIT SORBET
½ cup lemon sorbet or other fruit sorbet.

DAILY NUTRITION INFORMATION

1,345 calories

87 grams protein

157 grams carbohydrate

50 grams fat

26 grams fiber

DAY 11

BREAKFAST: PEACH-NUT OATMEAL
Cook ½ cup raw oats in 1 cup skim milk; when cooked, add ½ tsp cinnamon, 1 chopped peach and 2 tbsp chopped walnuts.

LUNCH: LENTIL SOUP AND SALAD
1 cup prepared lentil soup (approximately 200 calories) with mixed green salad composed of 2 cups mixed greens, 1 cup red and green pepper strips, ½ sliced cucumber, 5 cherry tomatoes and 2 tbsp slivered almonds. Dress salad with 2 tbsp light vinaigrette dressing and serve with 1 small orange.

SNACK: COOKIES AND MILK
2 graham cracker cookie squares and 1 cup skim milk.

DINNER: BROILED SALMON WITH STRING BEANS
Broil a 6-ounce salmon fillet with lemon juice and parsley (or herb of choice). Serve with sautéed string beans (sautéed in 1 tsp olive oil and minced garlic) and 1 small baked potato topped with 1 tsp butter.

EVENING SNACK: FRUIT AND YOGURT
½ cup sliced peach (or other fruit of choice) with ⅓ cup low-fat yogurt.

DAILY NUTRITION INFORMATION

1,328 calories

86 grams protein

150 grams carbohydrate

45 grams fat

26 grams fiber

DAY **12**

BREAKFAST: SCRAMBLED EGGS WITH SALSA
Whisk 1 egg yolk with 4 egg whites, then scramble them in a non-stick skillet with ¼ cup sliced white mushrooms. Pile eggs into ½ of a 6-inch whole-wheat pita pocket and add 1 to 2 tbsp jarred salsa. Serve with ½ medium grapefruit.

LUNCH: SPINACH SALAD
Pile 3 ounces sliced chicken breast, ¼ cup chopped red onion, 5 cherry tomatoes, ½ cup sliced cucumber, ½ cup sliced white mushrooms, ½ cup black beans and ½ cup chickpeas, onto a bed of fresh baby spinach leaves. Top the spinach salad with 2 tbsp grated Parmesan cheese and toss with 1 tsp olive oil plus vinegar and lemon to taste.

SNACK: ALMONDS AND APRICOTS
12 raw almonds and 4 dried apricot halves.

DINNER: WHOLE-WHEAT ZITI
Measure ¾ cup cooked whole-wheat ziti. Place hot ziti in an oven-proof bowl, top with ½ cup tomato sauce and ½ cup grated part-skim mozzarella cheese. Bake the pasta in the oven at 325° F for 10 to 15 minutes, or until the cheese is bubbly. Serve with salad (1 cup salad greens, ¼ cup chopped tomato, ¼ cup sliced cucumber and ¼ cup bell pepper) dressed with light vinaigrette dressing and 2 tbsp grated Parmesan cheese.

DAILY NUTRITION INFORMATION
1,326 calories
92 grams protein
147 grams carbohydrate
46 grams fat
34 grams fiber

EVENING SNACK: BERRIES AND CREAM
½ cup fresh mixed berries topped with 1 tsp non-dairy whipped cream.

DAY **13**

BREAKFAST: CEREAL AND MELON

In a bowl, mix ¾ cup high fiber cereal with 1 cup skim milk and 1 tbsp slivered almonds. Serve with 1 cup melon balls.

LUNCH: ROASTED VEGETABLES AND HUMMUS SANDWICH

Spread 2 tbsp hummus on 2 slices whole-grain bread and layer with 2 slices tomato and roasted red peppers (buy jarred roasted red peppers in brine) and slices of zucchini squash. Garnish the plate with ½ cup canned chickpeas and 10 baby carrots.

SNACK: PEANUT BUTTER CELERY STALKS

Fill 3 celery stalks with 2 tbsp all-natural peanut butter

DINNER: FLANK STEAK WITH SLICED TOMATO SALAD

Grill (or broil) 5 ounces of flank steak. When the steak is cooked to your liking, slice it thinly and top with 1 cup sliced mushrooms and onions sautéed in 1 tsp olive oil. Serve with steamed broccoli seasoned with fresh lemon juice and pepper. Serve with 1 medium size tomato and ¼ sliced cucumber salad, dressed with 2 tbsp light vinaigrette dressing.

EVENING SNACK: FRESH FRUIT

1 cup watermelon cubes.

DAILY NUTRITION INFORMATION

182 calories

83 grams protein

153 grams carbohydrate

45 grams fat

35 grams fiber

DAY **14**

BREAKFAST: BERRY-CINNAMON COTTAGE CHEESE
Combine 1 cup 1% cottage cheese with ½ cup fresh (or unsweetened frozen) mixed berries, 1 tsp ground cinnamon and 1 packet sweetener (if desired).

LUNCH: WHOLE-WHEAT PASTA SALAD
Toss ½ cup cooked whole-wheat pasta, 1 cup steamed assorted vegetables (such as broccoli, string beans, carrots, cauliflower), ½ cup canned white beans, 1 tsp olive oil, 1 tbsp chopped fresh herbs (such as basil or thyme) and 3 tbsp shredded Parmesan cheese. Serve chilled or warm (as desired).

SNACK: RICE CAKE AND PEANUT BUTTER
1 whole-grain rice cake spread with 2 tsp all-natural peanut butter.

DINNER: GREEK SALAD WITH GRILLED CHICKEN
In a large bowl, toss 4 to 5 ounces of grilled white meat chicken strips, ¼ cup crumbled feta cheese, 1 chopped tomato, ½ sliced cucumber, ½ cup chickpeas and ⅛ sliced avocado. Dress with 2 tbsp light vinaigrette dressing. Serve with ½ of a 6-inch whole-wheat pita.

EVENING SNACK: BAKED APPLE SLICES
Core and slice 1 medium apple. Place the apple slices in a baking dish and sprinkle with cinnamon. Cover and cook at 350° F for about 20 to 30 minutes. Enjoy warm with sweetener (if desired).

DAILY NUTRITION INFORMATION
1,293 calories
86 grams protein
140 grams carbohydrate
46 grams fat
30 grams fiber

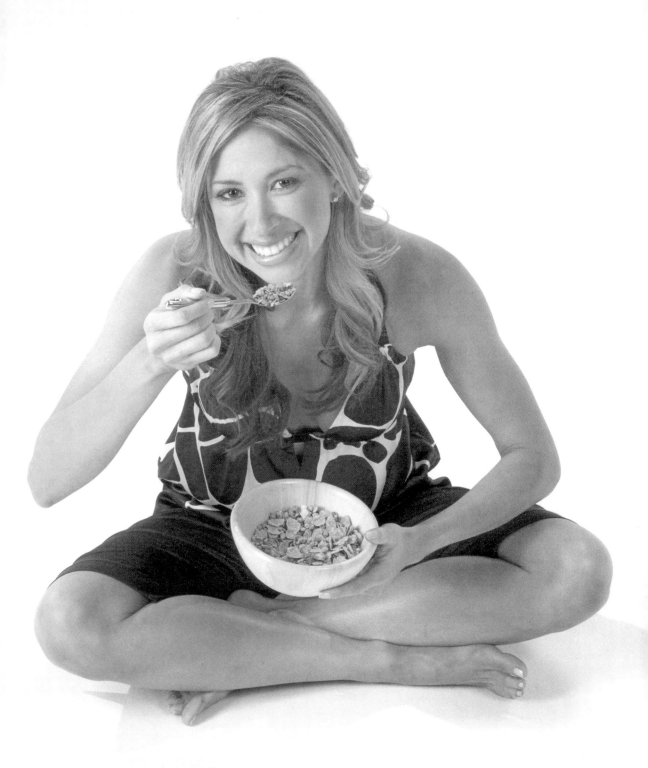

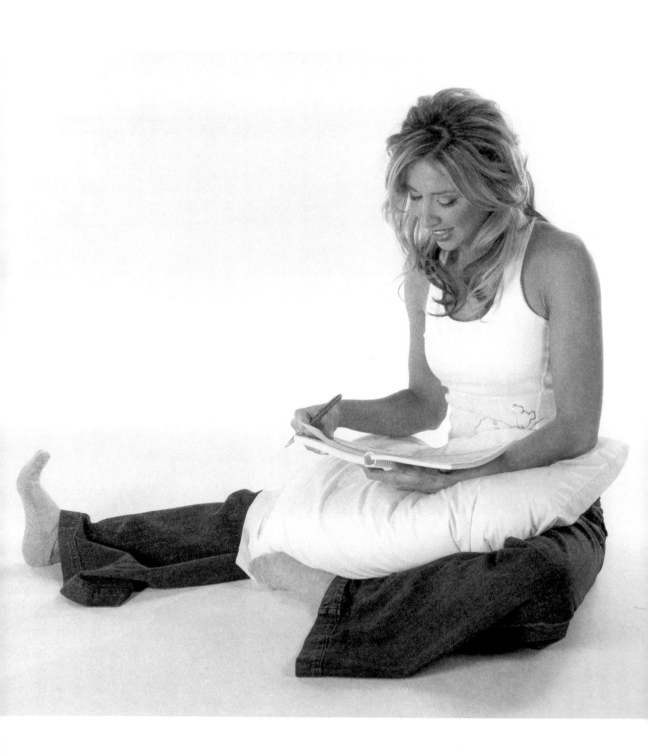

CHAPTER 7
PUTTING IT ALL TOGETHER

We know that for lasting results, small, gradual changes are key. The following pages are designed to help you get into the rhythm of exercising and eating right, step by step. Remember — the secret to success is finding the right program for you, one that delivers results that you can see and feel, and is do-able for you on a long-term basis.

STEP 1: SET GOALS

By setting specific goals, you'll give yourself something tangible to work toward, it will help you stay focused and motivated in the weeks and months ahead. Putting those goals in writing will help affirm your commitment and increase your chances for success. Use our worksheet to determine your long- and short-term goals, and record them in the spaces provided.

GOALS WORKSHEET

1. Start by identifying your long-term goals. Do you want to lose 20 pounds? Get stronger? Feel more energetic? Next, set a time frame for achieving those goals. For example, if your goal is to lose 20 pounds, try to estimate how long it realistically should take. For safe, lasting weight loss, you should aim to lose no more than 1 to 2 pounds a week. Remember: Your goals must be achievable; otherwise, you'll be setting yourself up for failure. So be sure to set your sights on a practical amount of weight to lose and a sensible time frame.

EXAMPLE:
My long-term fitness goals: Lose 20 pounds
My time frame: 20 weeks

2. Next, break your long-term goal into smaller short-term goals. For instance, if your goal is to lose 20 pounds in 20 weeks, break those 20 weeks up into five 4-week periods. Your first short-term goal will be to lose 4 pounds by the end of Week 4; your next goal will be to lose 8 pounds by the end of Week 8; and so on.

EXAMPLE:
My short-term fitness goal: Lose 4 pounds
My time frame: 4 weeks

YOUR GOALS

My long-term fitness goal: _____

My time frame: _____

Start date:

End date:

My short-term fitness goal: _____

My time frame: _____

Start date:

End date:

STEP 2: TAKE YOUR MEASUREMENTS

Nothing is more inspiring than noticing your clothes getting looser. That's why taking your measurements and stepping on the scale before getting started is important to see how much progress you've made. Once you know your starting measurements, you'll also be able to determine how effective your fitness and nutrition program is.

Grab a measuring tape: place it around the widest part of your chest, waist, hips and thighs. Take them first thing in the morning and don't wear thick clothing. Next, weigh yourself on a scale. (Note: When you weigh yourself again, you'll want to use the same scale.) Record your results in the spaces provided.

YOUR STARTING MEASUREMENTS

Date:

Chest   _____

Waist   _____

Hips   _____

Thighs   _____

Weight   _____

STEP 3: GET MOVING!

Dance cardio is one of the best workouts for trimming down because it burns lots of calories without putting stress on your joints. We've provided a few workout schedules for you depending on your fitness level that you previously determined in Chapter 2, Getting Started.

WEEKS 1–3 DANCE WORKOUT — BEGINNER

PERFORM 1 TIME PER WEEK; 30 MIN ROUTINE

This schedule has been designed to gently build you into a regular routine of dance cardio. For the first few weeks, you are going to perform this routine once a week, giving your body plenty of time to rest and recover. As you become more comfortable with the routine, you will be able to add extra steps and a faster beat to increase your workout intensity.

WARM-UP

MARCH	4 times (16 steps)
MARCH OUT WIDE	2 times (8 steps)
MARCH	1 time (4 steps)
MARCH OUT WIDE	1 time (4 steps out to the side)
MARCH	1 time (4 steps)
STEP TOUCH SIDE TO SIDE	4 times (16 steps)
TRAVEL UP	2 times (8 steps forward)
TRAVEL BACK	2 times (8 steps back)
STEP TOUCH SIDE TO SIDE	2 times (16 steps to the side)
TRAVEL UP	2 times (8 steps forward)
TRAVEL BACK	2 times (8 steps back)
STEP TOUCH SIDE TO SIDE	2 times (8 steps to the side)
STEP TOUCH SIDE TO SIDE LOW	2 times (8 steps to the side)
STEP TOUCH SIDE TO SIDE	2 times (8 steps to the side)
TRAVEL UP	2 times (8 steps forward)

STRETCH

SHOULDER SIDE TO SIDE	4 to the right, 4 to the left
SHOULDER ROLL	4 to the right, 4 to the left
PLIE	4 plies
PLIE ARMS TO THE FRONT	4 plies
HAMSTRING STRETCH	4 stretches to the right, 4 stretches to the left
WIDE LEG STRETCH	2 stretches
PIVOT STRETCH	2 pivots to the right, 2 pivots to the left
SHAKE AND SHIMEE	4 shakes to the right, 4 shakes to the left
SIDE TO SIDE STRETCH	4 to the right, 4 to the left
SHOULDER ROLL	4 rolls to the right, 4 rolls to the left

DANCE ROUTINE

MARCH UP AND BACK	4 times march up and back
MARCH	8 marches in place
RUNWAY STRUT	4 times up and back
MARCH	8 marches in place
SIDE TAP RIGHT	3 side taps to the right
RUNWAY STRUT	4 times up and back
SIDE TAP RIGHT	3 side taps to the right
MARCH IT BACK	1 time march back
RUNWAY STRUT	4 times up and back
SIDE TAP RIGHT	3 side taps to the right
MARCH IT BACK	1 time march back
MARCH	8 marches in place
MARCH IT UP AND BACK	2 times march up and back
SIDE TAP LEFT	3 side taps to the left
MARCH IT BACK	1 time march back
RUNWAY STRUT	4 times up and back
SIDE TAP LEFT	3 side taps to the left
MARCH IT UP	1 time march up
SIDE TAP LEFT	3 side taps to the left
MARCH IT BACK	1 time march back

SIDE TAP RIGHT	3 side taps to the right
MARCH IT BACK	1 time march back
MARCH IT UP	1 time march up
SIDE TAP LEFT	3 side taps to the left
MARCH IT BACK	1 time march back
SIDE TAP RIGHT	3 side taps to the right
MARCH IT BACK	1 time march back
MARCH	8 marches in place
MARCH IT UP AND BACK	2 times march up and back
STEP TOUCH SIDE TO SIDE	4 times to the right, 4 times to the left
MARCH	8 marches in place
STEP TOUCH SIDE TO SIDE ELONGATED	4 times to the right, 4 times to the left
STEP TOUCH SIDE TO SIDE	4 times to the right, 4 times to the left
STEP TOUCH SIDE TO SIDE ELONGATED	4 times to the right, 4 times to the left
STEP TOUCH SIDE TO SIDE	4 times to the right, 4 times to the left
STEP TOUCH SIDE TO SIDE ELONGATED	4 times to the right, 4 times to the left
GRAPEVINE	4 times to the right, 4 times to the left

COOL DOWN

ARMS UP	1 time
STEP TOUCH	4 times to the right, 4 times to the left
GRAPEVINE	1 time
STEP TOUCH	4 times to the right, 4 times to the left
GRAPEVINE	1 time to the right, 1 time to the left
STEP TOUCH	4 times to the right, 4 times to the left
GRAPEVINE	1 time
STEP TOUCH	4 times to the right, 4 times to the left
MARCH	1 time
MARCH OUT WIDE	1 time

ARMS UP	1 time
FLAT BACK DOWN	1 time
ROUND BACK UP	1 time
FLAT BACK DOWN	1 time
ROUND BACK UP	1 time
FLAT BACK DOWN	1 time
SINGLE ROUND BACK	4 times
RAGDOLL STRETCH	1 time
SHOULDER ROLL BACK	1 time
HIP ROCK UP	1 time
SHOULDER ROLL BACK	1 time
ARMS UP	1 time
HALF-MOON STRETCH	1 time
BALLET STRETCH	4 times (to the right, center and left)

WEEKS 1–3 DANCE WORKOUT — INTERMEDIATE/ADVANCED

PERFORM 2 TIMES PER WEEK; 35 MIN ROUTINE; WORK AT AN PRE OF 5

This schedule has been designed to get you back into the groove of doing regular cardio. For the first few weeks, you are going to perform this routine twice a week. As you quickly become more conditioned, you will be able to add extra combinations and additional steps to increase your workout intensity.

WARM-UP

MARCH	8 times
MARCH OUT WIDE	4 times
MARCH	2 times
MARCH OUT WIDE	2 times
MARCH	2 times

STEP TOUCH SIDE TO SIDE	2 times
TRAVEL UP	4 times
TRAVEL BACK	4 times
STEP TOUCH SIDE TO SIDE	4 times
TRAVEL UP	4 times
TRAVEL BACK	4 times
STEP TOUCH SIDE TO SIDE	4 times
STEP TOUCH SIDE TO SIDE LOW	4 times
STEP TOUCH SIDE TO SIDE	4 times
TRAVEL UP	4 times
TRAVEL BACK LOW	1 time
TRAVEL UP	1 time
TRAVEL BACK LOW	1 time
TRAVEL UP	1 time
TRAVEL BACK LOW	1 time

STRETCH

SHOULDER SIDE TO SIDE	4 to each side
SHOULDER ROLL	4 to the right, 4 to the left
PLIE	4 plies
PLIE ARMS TO THE FRONT	4 plies
HAMSTRING STRETCH	2 stretches to the right, 2 stretches to the left
WIDE LEG STRETCH	2 stretches
PIVOT STRETCH	2 pivots to the right, 2 pivots to the left
SHAKE AND SHIMEE	4 shakes to the right, 4 shakes to the left
SIDE TO SIDE STRETCH	4 to the right, 4 to the left
SHOULDER ROLL	4 rolls to the right, 4 rolls to the left

DANCE ROUTINE

MARCH IT UP AND BACK	4 times
MARCH	8 marches in place
RUNWAY STRUT	4 times up and back
MARCH	8 marches in place
SIDE TAP RIGHT	3 side taps to the right
RUNWAY STRUT	4 times up and back
SIDE TAP RIGHT	3 side taps to the right
MARCH IT BACK	1 time march back
RUNWAY STRUT	4 times up and back
SIDE TAP RIGHT	3 side taps to the right
MARCH IT BACK	1 time march back
MARCH	8 marches in place
MARCH IT UP AND BACK	2 times march up and back
SIDE TAP LEFT	3 side taps to the left
MARCH IT BACK	1 time march back
RUNWAY STRUT	4 times up and back
SIDE TAP LEFT	3 side taps to the left
MARCH IT UP	1 time march up
SIDE TAP LEFT	3 side taps to the left
MARCH IT BACK	1 time march back
SIDE TAP RIGHT	3 side taps to the right
MARCH IT BACK	1 time march back
MARCH IT UP	1 time march up
SIDE TAP LEFT	3 side taps to the left
MARCH IT BACK	1 time march back
SIDE TAP RIGHT	3 side taps to the right
MARCH IT BACK	1 time march back
MARCH	8 marches in place
MARCH IT UP AND BACK	2 times march up and back
STEP TOUCH SIDE TO SIDE	4 times to the right, 4 times to the left
MARCH	8 marches in place

STEP TOUCH SIDE TO SIDE ELONGATED	4 times to the right, 4 times to the left
STEP TOUCH SIDE TO SIDE	4 times to the right, 4 times to the left
STEP TOUCH SIDE TO SIDE ELONGATED	4 times to the right, 4 times to the left
STEP TOUCH SIDE TO SIDE BACK TOUCH	4 times to the right, 4 times to the left
STEP TOUCH SIDE TO SIDE ELONGATED	4 times to the right, 4 times to the left
GRAPEVINE	4 times to the right, 4 times to the left
CHEST POP	4 pops
GRAPEVINE RIGHT	1 time to the right
CHEST POP	4 pops
GRAPEVINE LEFT	1 time to the left
ELBOW HIGH POP	4 pops
GRAPEVINE RIGHT	1 time to the right
ELBOW HIGH POP	4 pops
GRAPEVINE LEFT	1 time to the left
ELBOW HIGH POP	4 pops
GRAPEVINE RIGHT	1 time to the right
ELBOW HIGH POP	4 pops
GRAPEVINE LEFT	1 time to the left
RUNWAY STRUT	1 time
STEP TOUCH SIDE	1 time to the left
MARCH IT BACK	1 time march back

COOL DOWN

ARMS UP	1 time
STEP TOUCH	4 times to the right, 4 times to the left
GRAPEVINE	1 time to the right, 1 time to the left
STEP TOUCH	4 times to the right, 4 times to the left
GRAPEVINE	1 time to the right, 1 time to the left

STEP TOUCH	4 times to the right, 4 times to the left
GRAPEVINE	1 time to the right, 1 time to the left
STEP TOUCH	4 times to the right, 4 times to the left
MARCH	1 time
MARCH WIDE	1 time
ARMS UP	1 time
FLAT BACK DOWN	1 time
ROUND BACK UP	1 time
FLAT BACK DOWN	1 time
ROUND BACK UP	1 time
FLAT BACK DOWN	1 time
SINGLE ROUND BACK	4 times
RAGDOLL STRETCH	1 time
SHOULDER ROLL BACK	1 time
HIP ROCK UP	1 time
SHOULDER ROLL BACK	1 time
ARMS UP	1 time
HALF-MOON STRETCH	1 time
BALLET STRETCH	4 times (to the right, center and left)

EXERCISE STATS:

Total time it took to perform the routine:

On a scale of 1 – 10, how hard did the routine feel to perform? Refer to the chart on page 28 for a refresher on using the scale.

How I felt immediately after the workout:

Changes I will make for the next workout: (Increase dance steps, find a bigger space to dance in, wear different clothing, etc)

My next workout will be on (date):

Use the talk test to determine if you are working hard enough — try reciting the alphabet or speak the lyrics to your favorite song aloud. If you can speak comfortably, then you're exercising at an appropriate intensity. If you have trouble breathing, you should slow down a bit.

WEEKS 4–6

Congratulations; you've come a long way! Now that you are used to the routines and are in the groove of working out on a regular basis, we've upped the ante with your exercise routines by adding an additional workout per week, as well as including new combinations and extra steps.

WEEKS 4–6 DANCE WORKOUT — BEGINNER
PERFORM 2 TIMES PER WEEK; 35 MIN ROUTINE; WORK AT AN PRE OF 5

WARM-UP

MARCH	8 times
MARCH OUT WIDE	4 times
MARCH	2 times
MARCH OUT WIDE	2 times
MARCH	2 times
STEP TOUCH SIDE TO SIDE	2 times
TRAVEL UP	4 times
TRAVEL BACK	4 times
STEP TOUCH SIDE TO SIDE	4 times
TRAVEL UP	4 times
TRAVEL BACK	4 times
STEP TOUCH SIDE TO SIDE	4 times
STEP TOUCH SIDE TO SIDE LOW	4 times
STEP TOUCH SIDE TO SIDE	4 times
TRAVEL UP	4 times
TRAVEL BACK LOW	1 time
TRAVEL UP	1 time
TRAVEL BACK LOW	1 time
TRAVEL UP	1 time
TRAVEL BACK LOW	1 time

STRETCH

SHOULDER SIDE TO SIDE	4 to each side
SHOULDER ROLL	4 to the right, 4 to the left
PLIE	4 plies
PLIE ARMS TO THE FRONT	4 plies
HAMSTRING STRETCH	2 stretches to the right, 2 stretches to the left
WIDE LEG STRETCH	2 stretches
PIVOT STRETCH	2 pivots to the right, 2 pivots to the left
SHAKE AND SHIMEE	4 shakes to the right, 4 shakes to the left
SIDE TO SIDE STRETCH	4 to the right, 4 to the left
SHOULDER ROLL	4 rolls to the right, 4 rolls to the left

DANCE ROUTINE

MARCH UP AND BACK	4 times
MARCH	8 marches in place
RUNWAY STRUT	4 times up and back
MARCH	8 marches in place
SIDE TAP RIGHT	3 side taps to the right
RUNWAY STRUT	4 times up and back
SIDE TAP RIGHT	3 side taps to the right
MARCH IT BACK	1 time march back
RUNWAY STRUT	4 times up and back
SIDE TAP RIGHT	3 side taps to the right
MARCH IT BACK	1 time march back
MARCH	8 marches in place
MARCH IT UP AND BACK	2 times march up and back
SIDE TAP LEFT	3 side taps to the left
MARCH IT BACK	1 time march back
RUNWAY STRUT	4 times up and back
SIDE TAP LEFT	3 side taps to the left
MARCH IT UP	1 time march up
SIDE TAP LEFT	3 side taps to the left

MARCH IT BACK	1 time march back
SIDE TAP RIGHT	3 side taps to the right
MARCH IT BACK	1 time march back
MARCH IT UP	1 time march up
SIDE TAP LEFT	3 side taps to the left
MARCH IT BACK	1 time march back
SIDE TAP RIGHT	3 side taps to the right
MARCH IT BACK	1 time march back
MARCH	8 marches in place
MARCH IT UP AND BACK	2 times march up and back
STEP TOUCH SIDE TO SIDE	4 times to the right, 4 times to the left
MARCH	8 marches in place
STEP TOUCH SIDE TO SIDE ELONGATED	4 times to the right, 4 times to the left
STEP TOUCH SIDE TO SIDE	4 times to the right, 4 times to the left
STEP TOUCH SIDE TO SIDE ELONGATED	4 times to the right, 4 times to the left
STEP TOUCH SIDE TO SIDE BACK TOUCH	4 times to the right, 4 times to the left
STEP TOUCH SIDE TO SIDE ELONGATED	4 times to the right, 4 times to the left
GRAPEVINE	4 times to the right, 4 times to the left
CHEST POP	4 pops
GRAPEVINE RIGHT	1 time to the right
CHEST POP	4 pops
GRAPEVINE LEFT	1 time to the left
ELBOW HIGH POP	4 pops
GRAPEVINE RIGHT	1 time to the right
ELBOW HIGH POP	4 pops
GRAPEVINE LEFT	1 time to the left
ELBOW HIGH POP	4 pops
GRAPEVINE RIGHT	1 time to the right

ELBOW HIGH POP	4 pops
GRAPEVINE LEFT	1 time to the left
RUNWAY STRUT	1 time
STEP TOUCH SIDE	1 time to the left
MARCH IT BACK	1 time march back

COOL DOWN

ARMS UP	1 time
STEP TOUCH	4 times to the right, 4 times to the left
GRAPEVINE	1 time to the right, 1 time to the left
STEP TOUCH	4 times to the right, 4 times to the left
GRAPEVINE	1 time to the right, 1 time to the left
STEP TOUCH	4 times to the right, 4 times to the left
GRAPEVINE	1 time to the right, 1 time to the left
STEP TOUCH	4 times to the right, 4 times to the left
MARCH	1 time
MARCH OUT WIDE	1 time
ARMS UP	1 time
FLAT BACK DOWN	1 time
ROUND BACK UP	1 time
FLAT BACK DOWN	1 time
ROUND BACK UP	1 time
FLAT BACK DOWN	1 time
SINGLE ROUND BACK	4 times
RAGDOLL STRETCH	1 time
SHOULDER ROLL BACK	1 time
HIP ROCK UP	1 time
SHOULDER ROLL BACK	1 time
ARMS UP	1 time
HALF-MOON STRETCH	1 time
BALLET STRETCH	4 times (to the right, center and left)

WEEKS 4–6 DANCE WORKOUT — INTERMEDIATE/ADVANCED

PERFORM 3 TIMES PER WEEK; 40 MIN ROUTINE; WORK AT AN PRE OF 6

Now that you are back in the groove, we've added one more dance session to your week for extra calorie burning.

WARM-UP

MARCH	8 times
MARCH OUT WIDE	4 times
MARCH	2 times
MARCH OUT WIDE	2 times
MARCH	2 times
STEP TOUCH SIDE TO SIDE	2 times
TRAVEL UP	4 times
TRAVEL BACK	4 times
STEP TOUCH SIDE TO SIDE	4 times
TRAVEL UP	4 times
TRAVEL BACK	4 times
STEP TOUCH SIDE TO SIDE	4 times
STEP TOUCH SIDE TO SIDE LOW	4 times
STEP TOUCH SIDE TO SIDE	4 times
TRAVEL UP	4 times
TRAVEL BACK LOW	1 time
TRAVEL UP	1 time
TRAVEL BACK LOW	1 time
TRAVEL UP	1 time
TRAVEL BACK LOW	1 time
STEP TOUCH	8 steps to the side
MARCH	8 steps in place
MARCH OUT WIDE	8 steps out to the side

ARMS UP STRETCH	2 times
LOOK SIDE TO SIDE	4 times
CHIN DOWN	4 times
CIRCLE NECK ROLLS	4 times
ARMS UP	1 time
FLAT BACK DOWN	3 times
ROUND BACK UP	3 times
SINGLE BACK	6 times
RAG DOLL STRETCH	1 time
ARMS UP	1 time

STRETCH

SHOULDER SIDE TO SIDE	4 to each side
SHOULDER ROLL	4 to the right, 4 to the left
PLIE	4 plies
PLIE ARMS TO THE FRONT	4 plies
HAMSTRING STRETCH	2 stretches to the right, 2 stretches to the left
WIDE LEG STRETCH	2 stretches
PIVOT STRETCH	2 pivots to the right, 2 pivots to the left
SHAKE AND SHIMEE	4 shakes to the right, 4 shakes to the left
SIDE TO SIDE STRETCH	4 to the right, 4 to the left
SHOULDER ROLL	4 rolls to the right, 4 rolls to the left

DANCE ROUTINE

MARCH IT UP AND BACK	4 marches
MARCH	8 marches in place
RUNWAY STRUT	4 times up and back
MARCH	8 marches in place
SIDE TAP RIGHT	3 side taps to the right
RUNWAY STRUT	4 times up and back
SIDE TAP RIGHT	3 side taps to the right
MARCH IT BACK	1 time march back

RUNWAY STRUT	4 times up and back
SIDE TAP RIGHT	3 side taps to the right
MARCH IT BACK	1 time march back
MARCH	8 marches in place
MARCH IT UP AND BACK	2 times
SIDE TAP LEFT	3 side taps to the left
MARCH IT BACK	1 time march back
RUNWAY STRUT	4 times up and back
SIDE TAP LEFT	3 side taps to the left
MARCH IT UP	1 time march up
SIDE TAP LEFT	3 side taps to the left
MARCH IT BACK	1 time march back
SIDE TAP RIGHT	3 side taps to the right
MARCH IT BACK	1 time march back
MARCH IT UP	1 time march up
SIDE TAP LEFT	3 side taps to the left
MARCH IT BACK	1 time march back
SIDE TAP RIGHT	3 side taps to the right
MARCH IT BACK	1 time march back
MARCH	8 marches in place
MARCH IT UP AND BACK	2 times
STEP TOUCH SIDE TO SIDE	4 times to the right, 4 times to the left
MARCH	8 marches in place
STEP TOUCH SIDE TO SIDE ELONGATED	4 times to the right, 4 times to the left
STEP TOUCH SIDE TO SIDE	4 times to the right, 4 times to the left
STEP TOUCH SIDE TO SIDE ELONGATED	4 times to the right, 4 times to the left
STEP TOUCH SIDE TO SIDE BACK TOUCH	4 times to the right, 4 times to the left
STEP TOUCH SIDE TO SIDE ELONGATED	4 times to the right, 4 times to the left

GRAPEVINE	4 times to the right, 4 times to the left
CHEST POP	4 pops
GRAPEVINE RIGHT	1 time to the right
CHEST POP	4 pops
GRAPEVINE LEFT	1 time to the left
ELBOW HIGH POP	4 pops
GRAPEVINE RIGHT	1 time to the right
ELBOW HIGH POP	4 pops
GRAPEVINE LEFT	1 time to the left
ELBOW HIGH POP	4 pops
GRAPEVINE RIGHT	1 time to the right
ELBOW HIGH POP	4 pops
GRAPEVINE LEFT	1 time to the left
RUNWAY STRUT UP	1 time
STEP TOUCH SIDE LEFT	1 time to the left
MARCH IT BACK	1 time

COOL DOWN

ARMS UP	1 time
STEP TOUCH	4 times to the right, 4 times to the left
GRAPEVINE	1 time to the right, 1 time to the left
STEP TOUCH	4 times to the right, 4 times to the left
GRAPEVINE	1 time to the right, 1 time to the left
STEP TOUCH	4 times to the right, 4 times to the left
GRAPEVINE	1 time to the right, 1 time to the left
STEP TOUCH	4 times to the right, 4 times to the left
MARCH	1 time
MARCH OUT WIDE	1 time
ARMS UP	1 time
FLAT BACK DOWN	1 time
ROUND BACK UP	1 time
FLAT BACK DOWN	1 time

ROUND BACK UP	1 time
FLAT BACK DOWN	1 time
SINGLE ROUND BACK	4 times
RAGDOLL STRETCH	1 time
SHOULDER ROLL BACK	1 time
HIP ROCK UP	1 time
SHOULDER ROLL BACK	1 time
ARMS UP	1 time
HALF-MOON STRETCH	1 time
BALLET STRETCH	4 times (to the right, center and left)

EXERCISE STATS:

Congratulations, you did it! By completing the first six weeks of this program, you've taken significant steps toward improving your health and developing good habits you can keep. But remember: to continue getting results, you need to stick with it!

Total time it took to perform the routine:
On a scale of 1 – 10, how hard did the routine feel to perform? Refer to the chart on page 28 for a refresher on using the scale.

How I felt immediately after the workout:
Changes I will make for the next workout: (Increase dance steps, find a bigger space to dance in, wear different clothing, etc)

My next workout will be on (date):

WEEKS 7 AND BEYOND— ADVANCED

By now you should have a pretty good feel for what works best for you in your day and exercise routines to keep you committed and consistent. We've included an advanced workout routine for those of you who are up to the challenge; if you are not there yet, don't worry! You will be soon. Also, read beyond for helpful hints and tips to keep you on track when the going gets tough.

WARM-UP

MARCH	8 times
MARCH OUT WIDE	4 times
MARCH	2 times
MARCH OUT WIDE	2 times
MARCH	2 times
STEP TOUCH SIDE TO SIDE	2 times
TRAVEL UP	4 times
TRAVEL BACK	4 times
STEP TOUCH SIDE TO SIDE	4 times
TRAVEL UP	4 times
TRAVEL BACK	4 times
STEP TOUCH SIDE TO SIDE	4 times
STEP TOUCH SIDE TO SIDE LOW	4 times
STEP TOUCH SIDE TO SIDE	4 times
TRAVEL UP	4 times
TRAVEL BACK LOW	1 time
TRAVEL UP	1 time
TRAVEL BACK LOW	1 time
TRAVEL UP	1 time
TRAVEL BACK LOW	1 time
STEP TOUCH	8 steps to the side
MARCH	8 steps in place
MARCH OUT WIDE	8 steps out to the side
ARMS UP STRETCH	2 times
LOOK SIDE TO SIDE	4 times
CHIN DOWN	4 times
CIRCLE NECK ROLLS	4 times
ARMS UP	1 time
FLAT BACK DOWN	3 times
ROUND BACK UP	3 times
SINGLE BACK	6 times

RAG DOLL STRETCH	1 time
ARMS UP	1 time
SHOULDER SIDE TO SIDE	4 to each side
SHOULDER ROLL	4 to the right, 4 to the left
PLIE	4 plies
PLIE ARMS TO THE FRONT	4 plies
HAMSTRING STRETCH	2 stretches to the right, 2 stretches to the left
WIDE LEG STRETCH	2 stretches
PIVOT STRETCH	2 pivots to the right, 2 pivots to the left
SHAKE AND SHIMEE	4 shakes to the right, 4 shakes to the left
SIDE TO SIDE STRETCH	4 to the right, 4 to the left
SHOULDER ROLL	4 rolls to the right, 4 rolls to the left

DANCE ROUTINE

MARCH IT UP AND BACK	4 marches
MARCH	8 marches in place
RUNWAY STRUT	4 times up and back
MARCH	8 marches in place
SIDE TAP RIGHT	3 side taps to the right
RUNWAY STRUT	4 times up and back
SIDE TAP RIGHT	3 side taps to the right
MARCH IT BACK	1 time march back
RUNWAY STRUT	4 times up and back
SIDE TAP RIGHT	3 side taps to the right
MARCH IT BACK	1 time march back
MARCH	8 marches in place
MARCH IT UP AND BACK	2 times
SIDE TAP LEFT	3 side taps to the left
MARCH IT BACK	1 time march back
RUNWAY STRUT	4 times up and back
SIDE TAP LEFT	3 side taps to the left
MARCH IT UP	1 time march up

SIDE TAP LEFT	3 side taps to the left
MARCH IT BACK	1 time march back
SIDE TAP RIGHT	3 side taps to the right
MARCH IT BACK	1 time march back
MARCH IT UP	1 time march up
SIDE TAP LEFT	3 side taps to the left
MARCH IT BACK	1 time march back
SIDE TAP RIGHT	3 side taps to the right
MARCH IT BACK	1 time march back
MARCH	8 marches in place
MARCH IT UP AND BACK	2 times
STEP TOUCH SIDE TO SIDE	4 times to the right, 4 times to the left
MARCH	8 marches in place
STEP TOUCH SIDE TO SIDE ELONGATED	4 times to the right, 4 times to the left
STEP TOUCH SIDE TO SIDE	4 times to the right, 4 times to the left
STEP TOUCH SIDE TO SIDE ELONGATED	4 times to the right, 4 times to the left
STEP TOUCH SIDE TO SIDE BACK TOUCH	4 times to the right, 4 times to the left
STEP TOUCH SIDE TO SIDE ELONGATED	4 times to the right, 4 times to the left
GRAPEVINE	4 times to the right, 4 times to the left
CHEST POP	4 pops
GRAPEVINE RIGHT	1 time to the right
CHEST POP	4 pops
GRAPEVINE LEFT	1 time to the left
ELBOW HIGH POP	4 pops
GRAPEVINE RIGHT	1 time to the right
ELBOW HIGH POP	4 pops
GRAPEVINE LEFT	1 time to the left
ELBOW HIGH POP	4 pops

GRAPEVINE RIGHT	1 time to the right
ELBOW HIGH POP	4 pops
GRAPEVINE LEFT	1 time to the left
RUNWAY STRUT UP	1 time
STEP TOUCH SIDE LEFT	1 time left
MARCH IT BACK	1 time
STEP TOUCH SIDE LEFT	1 time left
GRAPEVINE LEFT	1 time to the left
ELBOW HIGH POP	1 pop
GRAPEVINE RIGHT	1 time to the right
ELBOW HIGH POP	1 pop
RUNWAY STRUT UP	1 time up
SIDE TAP RIGHT	1 time to the right
MARCH IT BACK	1 time
SIDE TAP RIGHT	1 side tap to the right
GRAPEVINE RIGHT	1 time to the right
ELBOW HIGH POP	1 pop
GRAPEVINE LEFT	1 time to the left
ELBOW HIGH POP	1 pop
RUNWAY STRUT UP	1 time up
STEP TOUCH SIDE LEFT	1 time left
GRAPEVINE LEFT	1 time to the left
ELBOW HIGH POP	1 pop
GRAPEVINE RIGHT	1 time to the right
ELBOW HIGH POP	1 pop
RUNWAY STRUT UP	1 time up
SIDE TAP RIGHT	1 side tap to the right
MARCH IT BACK	1 time
SIDE TAP RIGHT	1 side tap to the right
GRAPEVINE RIGHT	1 time to the right
ELBOW HIGH POP	1 pop
GRAPEVINE LEFT	1 time to the left

ELBOW HIGH POP	1 pop
RUNWAY STRUT UP	1 time up
CHEST POPS	4 pops
STEP TOUCH SIDE TO SIDE	4 times to the right, 4 times to the left
SIDE TO SIDE STOMP	4 times to the right, 4 times to the left
STEP TOUCH SIDE TO SIDE	4 times to the right, 4 times to the left
STEP TOUCH SIDE TO SIDE	
WITH SINGLE ARM ROW	4 times to the right, 4 times to the left
SIDE TO SIDE STOMP	4 times to the right, 4 times to the left
STEP STOP RIGHT	8 times to the right
BOUNCE	2 bounces
STEP STOP	8 times to the left
BOUNCE	2 bounces
STEP STOP RIGHT	8 times to the right
BOUNCE	2 bounces
STEP STOP LEFT	8 times to the left
BOUNCE	2 bounces
STEP STOP RIGHT	8 times to the right
BOUNCE	2 bounces
STEP TOUCH SIDE TO SIDE	1 time to the right, 1 time to the left
SNAKE RIGHT	2 times to the right
SNAKE LEFT	2 times to the left
SNAKE RIGHT	2 times to the right
SNAKE LEFT	2 times to the left
STEP TOUCH SIDE TO SIDE	2 times to the right, 2 times to the left
TRAVEL UP	1 time
STEP TOUCH SIDE TO SIDE	2 times to the right, 2 times to the left
TRAVEL BACK	1 time
SNAKE UP	2 steps forward
SNAKE BACK	2 steps back
SNAKE UP	2 steps forward
SNAKE BACK	2 steps back

SNAKE UP	2 steps forward
SNAKE BACK	2 steps back
SNAKE UP	2 steps forward
SNAKE BACK	2 steps back
SNAKE RIGHT	2 times to the right
SNAKE LEFT	2 times to the left
SNAKE RIGHT	2 times to the right
SNAKE LEFT	2 times to the left
SNAKE UP	2 steps forward
SNAKE BACK	2 steps back
SNAKE UP	2 steps forward
SNAKE BACK	2 steps back
STEP TOUCH SIDE TO SIDE	2 times to the right, 2 times to the left
SWIM	2 times to the right, 2 times to the left (8 times)
STEP STOMP SIDE TO SIDE	4 times to the right, 4 times to the left
KICK TAP BACK RIGHT LEG	4 times to the center
KICK KICK TAP BACK RIGHT LEG	4 times to the right corner
KICK TAP BACK RIGHT LEG	4 times to the left corner
DOUBLE BOUNCE	4 bounces
KICK TAP BACK LEFT LEG	4 times to the center
KICK KICK TAP BACK LEFT LEG	4 times to the left corner
KICK TAP BACK RIGHT LEG	4 times to the left corner
DOUBLE BOUNCE	4 bounces
TRIPLE STEP RIGHT LEAD LEG	2 times
DOUBLE BOUNCE	4 bounces
TRIPLE STEP LEFT LEAD LEG	4 times
DOUBLE BOUNCE	4 bounces
TRIPLE STEP RIGHT LEAD LEG	4 times
DOUBLE BOUNCE	4 bounces
TRIPLE STEP LEFT LEAD LEG	4 times
STEP TOUCH SIDE TO SIDE	2 times to the right, 2 times to the left

HIP HOP MOVE SIDE TO SIDE	8 times
STEP TOUCH SIDE TO SIDE	2 times to the right, 2 times to the left
HIP HOP MOVE SIDE TO SIDE	8 times
STEP TOUCH SIDE TO SIDE	2 times to the right, 2 times to the left
SCISSOR BOUNCE	4 times to the right, 4 times to the left
STEP TOUCH SIDE TO SIDE	2 times to the right, 2 times to the left
SCISSOR BOUNCE	4 times to the right, 4 times to the left
STEP TOUCH SIDE TO SIDE	2 times to the right, 2 times to the left
STEP TOUCH SIDE TO SIDE ELONGATED	8 times to the right, 8 times to the left
HIP ROCK SIDE TO SIDE	8 times to the right, 8 times to the left
STEP TOUCH SIDE TO SIDE BACK	8 times to the right, 8 times to the left
HIP ROCK SIDE TO SIDE	8 times to the right, 8 times to the left
RUNWAY UP AND BACK	1 time
HIP ROCK SIDE TO SIDE	8 times to the right, 8 times to the left
CIRCLE ARMS	8 times to the right, 8 times to the left
RUNWAY UP AND BACK	1 time
HIP ROCK SIDE TO SIDE	8 times to the right, 8 times to the left
CIRCLE ARMS	2 times to the right, 2 times to the left (4 times)
RUNWAY UP AND BACK	1 time
HIP ROCK SIDE TO SIDE	8 times to the right, 8 times to the left
COWGIRL CIRCLE AROUND THE WORLD *(4 times to the right)*	
HIP POP	12 times in place
RUNWAY UP AND BACK	1 time
HIP ROCK SIDE TO SIDE	8 times to the right, 8 times to the left
COWGIRL CIRCLE AROUND THE WORLD	4 times to the left
HIP POP	12 times in place
MARCH	1 time
HIP ROCK SIDE TO SIDE	8 times to the right, 8 times to the left
RUNWAY STRUT	1 time up and back

HIP ROCK SIDE TO SIDE	8 times to the right, 8 times to the left
RUNWAY STRUT	1 time up and back
CIRCLE ARMS	2 times to the right, 2 times to the left (4 times)
STRAIGHT LEGS HIP BOUNCE	16 times
HIP ROCK SIDE TO SIDE	8 times to the right, 8 times to the left
MARCH	1 time
MAMBO CHA CHA CHA	4 times to the right, 4 times to the left
BOX STEP RIGHT	12 times to the right
CHA CHA CHA	1 time
BOX STEP LEFT	12 times to the left
CHA CHA CHA	1 time
BOX STEP RIGHT	8 times to the right
CHA CHA CHA	1 time
BOX STEP LEFT	8 times to the left
CHA CHA CHA	1 time
BOX STEP RIGHT	8 times to the right
MAMBO CHA CHA CHA	1 time
MARCH	1 time
MAMBO FRONT	4 times to the right, 4 times to the left
MAMBO TO THE SIDE	4 times to the right
MAMBO TO THE SIDE	4 times to the left
STEP BACK WITH HEAD TURN	8 times to the right, 8 times to the left
MAMBO	1 time
KICK, CROSS, TOUCH	12 times, alternating
SHAKE AND SHIMMEE BACK	1 time
MAMBO	1 time
STEP BACK WITH HEAD TURN	8 times to the right, 8 times to the left
KICK, CROSS, TOUCH	12 times, alternating
SHAKE AND SHIMMEE BACK	1 time
DIAGONAL PUMP	2 times to the right, 2 times to the left
HEEL TAPS FRONT	4 times front

HEEL TAPS RIGHT	4 times to the right
HEEL TAPS BACK	4 times back
HEEL TAPS LEFT	4 times to the left
NEW SHOES FRONT	4 times front
NEW SHOES RIGHT	4 times to the right
NEW SHOES BACK	4 times back
NEW SHOES LEFT	4 times to the left
HOUSE IT WITH HIP TURN	4 times to the right, 4 times to the left
NOODLE LEGS CLOSE	8 times
NOODLE LEGS WIDE	8 times
CHEST BOUNCES	12 times in place
DIAGONAL PUMP	2 times to the right, 2 times to the left
STEP TOUCH SIDE TO SIDE	4 times to the right, 4 times to the left

COOL DOWN

ARMS UP	1 time
STEP TOUCH	4 times to the right, 4 times to the left
GRAPEVINE	1 time to the right, 1 time to the left
STEP TOUCH	4 times to the right, 4 times to the left
GRAPEVINE	1 time to the right, 1 time to the left
STEP TOUCH	4 times to the right, 4 times to the left
GRAPEVINE	1 time to the right, 1 time to the left
STEP TOUCH	4 times to the right, 4 times to the left
MARCH	1 time
MARCH OUT WIDE	1 time
ARMS UP	1 time
FLAT BACK DOWN	1 time
ROUND BACK UP	1 time
FLAT BACK DOWN	1 time
ROUND BACK UP	1 time
FLAT BACK DOWN	1 time
SINGLE ROUND BACK	4 times

RAGDOLL STRETCH	1 time
SHOULDER ROLL BACK	1 time
HIP ROCK UP	1 time
SHOULDER ROLL BACK	1 time
ARMS UP	1 time
HALF-MOON STRETCH	1 time
BALLET STRETCH	4 times (to the right, center and left)

STAYING ON TRACK

It's likely that at some point during the course of your exercise career, you'll run into the exercise doldrum, or will miss a few workout sessions due to reasons beyond your control. Don't let a few missed sessions or boredom stop the positive momentum of consistent exercise. Here are some tips to help keep the spark in your workouts.

TIP 1. ADD SOME STRENGTH WORK TO YOUR WORKOUT

As we get older, our muscles and bones get weaker, especially if we don't eat right or get enough physical activity. Regular strength training (exercising using weights or other resistance) can help prevent such losses to reduce your risk of bone fractures, back pain and other ailments. Even more exciting, it can help keep excess body fat at bay. When you build muscle, your metabolism speeds up, so you burn more calories all day long. Muscle weighs more than fat, but takes up less space, so even if the numbers on the scale don't change dramatically, your clothes will get looser, and your body will look firmer.

Try alternating theses exercises with your Dance Cardio Workout:

COUNTERTOP PUSH-UP

Place your hands on a countertop, shoulder-width apart. Keeping your arms straight, walk your feet back until your hips and back are straight, feet together. Lift up on the balls of your feet and bend your elbows to slowly lower your torso toward the countertop, until you're about six inches away. Slowly push back up to starting position, then repeat. Perform 10 times. Works chest, shoulders and triceps (back of arms).

CHAIR SQUAT

Stand 12 inches in front of a sturdy chair, then turn and face away from it, feet shoulder-width apart. Raise your arms in front of you to shoulder height. Bend your knees and slowly lower your buttocks down and back toward the chair, leaning forward slightly with your torso for balance. Once you feel the chair beneath you, straighten your legs, pushing up through your feet, to lift your body back up to starting position. Repeat 10 times. Works lower back, buttocks, legs.

HIP HINGE

Stand with your feet shoulder-width apart, hands on your hips. Keeping your knees straight and bending from your hips, lean forward until you feel a slight pull in the back of your legs. Slowly lift your torso to return to starting position. Repeat 10 times. Works your lower back, buttocks and hamstrings (back of thighs).

FLOOR CRUNCH

Lying on your back on the floor, bend your knees and place your feet flat on the floor, hip-width apart. Keeping your neck and back relaxed, cross your arms over your chest, resting each hand on opposite sides of your collarbone. Placing your chin on your wrists, position your elbows so they are pointing towards your knees. Lift your upper body up and towards your knees, exhaling, so that your shoulder blades come up off the ground. Once your shoulder blades have left the ground pause, then slowly return to the floor to begin another rep. Repeat 10 times. Works your abdominals.

Remember: keep your back relaxed and in contact with the floor through the entire exercise. Be sure to "pull" with your abs and not your neck.

KEEP AN EYE ON YOUR PROGRESS

Tape and weight measurements aren't the only indicators of how well you are doing on your exercise journey. Take a minute to think about how you feel: Do you have more energy? How are your hunger levels? Do you feel better about yourself? Remember, how you feel physically and mentally is just as important as how many pounds and inches you lose!

STAY MOTIVATED!

Studies show that most people need to stay with a habit for 30 to 60 days before their commitment takes hold. Here, four stick-with-it strategies to help you remain on track.

FIGURE OUT THE HOWS AND WHENS

If you fail to plan, you plan to fail. Make sure to sit down once a week to schedule your workouts for the next seven days with a specific time, location and routine. Treat them as important appointments that can't be missed.

Turn to page 156 to make photocopies of our Fitness Log to use in your planning.

DON'T THINK "ALL OR NOTHING"

If you miss a workout or eat something unhealthy, don't give up! Remember, your success lies in your ability to enact your plan over the long haul, not just today. If you have a bad day, you haven't blown it. So, pick yourself up and get back on track. It is very difficult to adhere to a fitness plan 100% the time — even with best preparation and planning.

BELIEVE THAT CHANGE IS POSSIBLE

Stop thinking that what you are setting out to do is impossible. It's easy to feel as if you don't have control over your life — believe that you can achieve your goals, as they are within your control, and you will make it happen.

REWARD YOURSELF

At the end of the day, the bottom line is that you are doing something positive and healthy for the most important person in your life — you. Once in a while, take the time to acknowledge your hard-earned commitment by rewarding yourself with a new workout outfit, CD or manicure. Being nice to yourself once in a while can keep your enthusiasm up and help to reinforce your newly-found healthy habits.

DAILY MEAL PLAN SHEET

MONDAY	TUESDAY	WEDNESDAY	THURSDAY
Breakfast	Breakfast	Breakfast	Breakfast
Lunch	Lunch	Lunch	Lunch
Snack	Snack	Snack	Snack
Dinner	Dinner	Dinner	Dinner
Snack	Snack	Snack	Snack
Water	Water	Water	Water
Comments	Comments	Comments	Comments

FRIDAY	SATURDAY	SUNDAY
Breakfast	Breakfast	Breakfast
Lunch	Lunch	Lunch
Snack	Snack	Snack
Dinner	Dinner	Dinner
Snack	Snack	Snack
Water	Water	Water
Comments	Comments	Comments

FITNESS LOG

DAY:

DATE:

WARM-UP

EXERCISE	X TO REPEAT	RIGHT/LEFT

WORKOUT

EXERCISE	X TO REPEAT	RIGHT/LEFT

EXERCISE	X TO REPEAT	RIGHT/LEFT

COOL DOWN

EXERCISE	X TO REPEAT	RIGHT/LEFT

WEIGHT-LOSS, BODY-COMPOSITION AND BODY CIRCUMFERENCE SHEET

WEIGHT-LOSS AND BODY-COMPOSITION LOG

STARTING WEEK _____   DATE:

WEIGHT	BF %	LEAN MASS (LBS)	FAT MASS (LBS)

MY GOAL: _____   _____   _____   _____

WEEK _____   DATE:

WEIGHT	BF %	LEAN MASS (LBS)	FAT MASS (LBS)

CHANGE: _____   _____   _____   _____

WEEK _____   DATE:

WEIGHT	BF %	LEAN MASS (LBS)	FAT MASS (LBS)

CHANGE: _____   _____   _____   _____

WEEK _____   DATE:

WEIGHT	BF %	LEAN MASS (LBS)	FAT MASS (LBS)

WEIGHT-LOSS AND BODY-CIRCUMFERENCE LOG

STARTING WEEK _____   DATE: WEIGHT:

CHEST	MID-SECTION	HIPS	THIGHS

MY GOAL: _____   _____   _____   _____

WEEK _____   DATE: WEIGHT:

CHEST	MID-SECTION	HIPS	THIGHS

CHANGE: _____   _____   _____   _____

WEEK _____   DATE: WEIGHT:

CHEST	MID-SECTION	HIPS	THIGHS

CHANGE: _____   _____   _____   _____

WEEK _____   DATE: WEIGHT:

CHEST	MID-SECTION	HIPS	THIGHS

CHANGE: _____   _____   _____   _____